Undulation:

Relieve Stiffness
and Feel Young

Undulation: Relieve Stiffness and Feel Young

Second Edition

Author: Anita Boser

Foreword: Mary Bond

Introduction: Roger Golten

Photographer: Michael Boser

Designer: Jeanie James

The contents of this text are not meant to substitute for medical diagnosis or treatment of any kind. The author and publisher encourage the reader to consult with a qualified healthcare professional to determine their special fitness needs.

ISBN-13: 978-0-9796179-4-2

Library of Congress Control Number: 2016917417

    1. Health   2. Exercise

Undulation: Relieve Stiffness and Feel Young

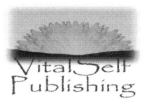

Table of Contents

Foreword

The process of aging, as most people experience it, involves a gradual diminishment of the ease and grace of movement. When we were children, free to improvise and play, our bodies expressed our curiosity about the world, and about our place in it, with Gumby-like adaptability. As we stepped into adulthood and became focused on careers, responsibilities, and roles, our relationship with the world began to require less and less bodily movement. In biomechanical terms, this meant that fewer of our joints were involved in the repetitive activities of the daily grind. Our joints became inhibited by restricted fascia—the body-wide and all-encompassing constitutive tissue of our bodies.

By age fifty, most of us will have given up attempting the games and dances that gave us pleasure when we were younger. Yet, as we contemplate our own aging, few of us identify with the stiff-looking movements of the elderly. What we observe in them is loss of fascial resilience. Fascia dehydrates and loses elasticity when deprived of the bodily movements that circulate fluids through it. Without attention to reversing this process by cultivating innovative movement, we too will likely complain of feeling stiffer and stiffer as the years go by.

Articulate joint mobility and free fascial tissue glide facilitate the effortless grace we admire in elite athletes and dancers. When the body's movement is restricted, a host of problems ensue. Restricted joints inhibit the coordination of muscles and interfere with the sequencing of movement. This, in turn, blocks the flow of nourishing fluids throughout the body. The resulting tissue dehydration can interfere with organ function and give rise to the so-called diseases of aging.

In *Undulation: Relieve Stiffness and Feel Young*, Anita Boser skillfully guides you through a program of innovative movement designed to restore the natural undulate flows in your body. By drawing your awareness to unconsciously restricted regions of your body, Anita guides you, step-by-step, into recovering lost joint function. The restored range of movement in your body will result in new opportunities for self-expression. By following her advice, you will refresh your spirit as well as reawaken your body.

> Mary Bond, MA
> Rolf Movement® Faculty,
> Rolf Institute® of Structural Integration, Boulder, CO
> Author of *The New Rules of Posture, Balancing Your Body, Heal Your Posture* (a DVD workshop), and *Your Body Mandala*.

Introduction

Think about all the different activities where spinal flexibility is essential. Without this flexibility it's very difficult to function fully in the world. Things like putting on your socks or tying your shoelaces, lying down, sitting and standing, looking behind you while reversing the car, or even dancing are difficult without flexibility.

Backache, stiffness, and pain are often associated with compression of the spinal vertebrae and the loss of hydration in the intervertebral discs. Without movement, there is stagnation, calcification, and dehydration, and the ability to move is lost—leading to more stagnation and less movement. It's a vicious circle.

The sedentary society has a lot to answer for. In the world in which many of us live, sitting has become one of our most common activities. We sit to eat; sit in the train or the car; sit at work; sit to watch TV and movies and interact with computers; and sit at home because we are tired of sitting all day! The price we are paying has been high in terms of health issues. Our bodies did not evolve to sit. We can learn to sit well or badly – most of us sit badly and then need to spend time rehabilitating with various kinds of exercise.

Fortunately, there is a counterbalancing trend of which this book is a part. The progressive nature of the approach outlined in the following pages can take you, wherever you have ended up on the journey of life, into a gentle exploration of your own body, and lead you forward to recovering mobility. But, before you do anything, it has to be mentally conceived, thought about, considered by the mind/body continuum.

If undulation is a new concept for you, please give yourself permission to master it gradually. Just thinking about and visualizing undulation is a valuable and important stage in the process of fluidizing your system. Human beings have a special relationship with water which is the essence of fluidity. We come from water and depend on it for healthy functioning.

Undulation also acknowledges the essential unity of the human system. We are not just a collection of parts—some of which work better than others. Undulation is a whole body movement. Everything is connected and affected by movement, and we are organised structures operating in and organised by gravity.

Loss of muscular tone is another main issue arising from our sedentary society. Hence the popularity and success of core stability exercise such as Pilates and the use of exercise balls. But you can undulate anywhere, anytime—sitting, standing, walking, lying on your side or front or in water. The best thing of all—it's fun!

Roger Golten
Hellerwork® Structural Integration Practitioner
& Shaw Method® swimming teacher
Author of *The Owner's Guide to the Body*

Dedicated to

The many people who have been willing to try something new and therefore were able to benefit from undulation.

Sway Every Day.

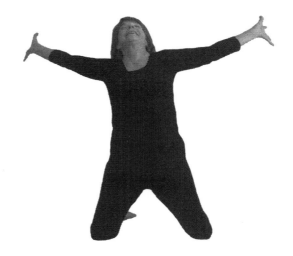

Chapter One

How to Get the Most out of

Undulation

THERE ARE AN INFINITE NUMBER OF WAYS TO MOVE, and there are an infinite number of reasons to move more. Feeling great, avoiding injury, and healing quickly—just like we did when we were kids—are some of the most common incentives, but the advantages extend beyond the physical realm. Moving more is good for the brain, and experiencing new freedom through movement allows for emotional and spiritual release as well.

Undulation will help you to diminish stiffness, whether you wake up with it each morning or just get sore after activity. In addition, undulation improves athletic performance, increases body intelligence, develops underused muscles, creates flexibility, and helps you move more easily and effortlessly.

1

When I wrote the first edition of this book in 2007, I knew that undulation helped many people feel good. Since then, I have learned more about why undulation is so effective. It is because it works on many levels at once.

- ❧ The human body is designed for a variety of movement. Undulation teaches you how to create variety on a regular basis rather than getting stuck in the rut of repetitive strain.

- ❧ We are more likely to get injured when we are in unfamiliar positions. Undulation gives the brain a chance to experience out-of-the-ordinary postures and develop intelligence and strength in those positions.

- ❧ It is optimal to improve range of motion before developing strength. Stretching can develop strength at the end ranges, but it isn't so good for the "nooks and crannies." Undulation is.

- ❧ There is an inverse relationship between how much your brain interprets sensations as pain (nociception) and how much your brain understands where your body is in space (proprioception and interoception). Undulation improves proprioception and interoception, and therefore reduce pain.

- ❧ After injury, sometimes the nervous system misinterprets signals and tells muscles to contract when they don't need to, but if the joint can rest where it was injured and come out of this position slowly, the nervous system gets a chance to reset the signal. When you learn to let your body lead undulations, it will often find these positions—and relief.

Based on feedback from the first edition, I have reorganized the information to make it easier for readers to find the undulations that will be most helpful. Each section includes four to six exercises, which together take from five to fifteen minutes, something feasible for most people on most days.

- ❧ The Fundamentals are good for everyone, anytime to improve your baseline spinal flexibility and body awareness.

- ❧ The other undulations are now categorized for where they are most effective: Low Back & Hips, Neck, Shoulders & Arms, Core Strength, Posture, and more.

- ❧ However, anyone will benefit from any undulation—as long as you follow the "no pain" guidelines on the next page. Even if you don't have low back pain, you will benefit from and probably enjoy Happy Dog. Even if you don't have scoliosis, your body will build strength and intelligence from the Mermaid (which is my favorite). Tailbone Penmanship is a favorite of most people, and I put it in the To Counteract Aging section.

I suggest doing the Fundamentals every other day and a section that appeals to you on the other days. When you are short on time, devote a minute or less to each one. On the days when you have more time or when your body is in particular need, you can extend your undulation time to a half an hour. Of course, you can build undulation into your daily activities, rather than setting aside time for it, too. (We even created a computer program called Undulation Break to remind people to undulate.)

Your body knows what it needs to feel better. The undulations will teach you how to listen to what it's saying. If you do the exercises in this book regularly, you'll become your own undulation expert—able to glide articulate, and flow. You'll feel younger and more alive.

The No-Pain Guidelines

The Most Important Part of This Book!

Pain signals that something is wrong. If you've ignored your body for long, pain may be the only way that it can communicate with you. Pay attention to the message and you'll cultivate the innate ability to hear what your body is saying.

Listen closely and notice. How do you feel when you undulate? Do you feel tension? Pleasure? Jerky or luxurious? How about relieved? Weird? Relaxed, stiff, joyful? Maybe nothing at all? All of these are OK.

Feeling pain is definitely not OK.

If a movement causes you pain, STOP! Back up and do the movement up to, but stopping short of, when it began to hurt. Try some variations. Move less, smaller or slower—whatever it takes to avoid the pain. If you can continue to move without discomfort, your tissues will be getting exactly what they need to heal. Eventually the pain-free range will increase.

How do you tell the difference between the pain caused by regular physical labor and that caused by internal injury? A weak muscle might feel painful while building up strength, but the pain should stop when the work stops. You may end up with a little soreness, but not a lasting ache. Injured muscles and tissues, however, will continue to feel pain long after exertion ends. Until you can easily tell the difference, avoid any movements that cause pain or discomfort.

If you are already feeling the stiffness of immobility, be extra-sensible with this program. Be mindful and please remember: injury can create scar tissue, and scar tissue can further restrict movement. As with any new exercise, I recommend that you discuss undulation with your physician before you begin. Take this book with you, so that you can show your doctor the movements involved.

> CAUTION: If you have osteoporosis, a currently diagnosed bulging disc, spondylosis, spondylolisthesis, or spinal stenosis, it is particularly important to review the exercises in this book with your doctor or physical therapist before you begin. People with these conditions must be very careful with flexion and extension (forward and backbending). Very slow and small movements can sometimes be tolerated, but I encourage you to get your personal health care provider's advice on this subject.

Getting Started

As you move through the material, you'll see that each section offers a wide variety of movement patterns. If some of the beginning exercises feel difficult, your body may have closed off that particular physical action. But it's nothing to lose any sleep over. You can regain the movements with continued practice. Also, there are no requirements that each undulation be perfect before moving on to the next one.

It's fine to skip around in the book to try out exercises that appeal to you rather than going in order. Be careful though that you're not missing an entire movement pattern. The power of undulation is in recreating lost motion. You undermine your success when you disregard exercises that target a particular portion of your spine or way of moving.

Breathe

Breath is fundamental to your body's fluid movement. Let your breath work within your muscles like a gentle massage to help you open up blockages. Keep your breathing relaxed and direct it into the areas that seem stuck. If you find your breath starts to feel restricted or that you've forgotten to breathe altogether, take a short break, because holding your breath prevents positive change.

Set Realistic Expectations

I was taught that my brain was the boss (and a pretty critical one at that!) and that my body was the (sometimes begrudging) servant.

Undulation can help you to establish a better mind-body balance. When you're able to mentally observe your undulations without judgment, the physical self will respond positively. Imagine the feelings that you'd like your body to know. Visualize water, warmth, or light flowing through your muscles. Use whatever feels, sounds, or looks right to you.

If you get discouraged because you're not performing as well as you'd like, stop for a moment. Relax and take a breath. As you exhale, focus on letting your frustration flow out with your breath. Whenever you start to feel that tension, take a breather. Forcing only creates rigidity.

If you undulate regularly, instead of your brain directing every movement, your spine may ultimately lead itself. Eventually, you may only need this book as a fun resource to return to if your daily undulations become stale.

There is no one, right way to undulate. It is ALL an exploration. The key to being more youthful is to continually add variety to your movements. And trying is actually more important than getting it. When you run across one of those "Argh, I can't do it," exercises, take heart. Recognize it as one that will probably be beneficial for you.

All types of movements are good. Jerky movements can create smoother ones. Irregular movements will lead to more even ones. Wobbly ones can build better balance.

Your goal is to regain movement and fluidity where it hasn't been, not to create a lot of movement in any one place. What might feel stiff or weird at first will become more comfortable as your connective tissues re-hydrate, muscles rebuild lost strength, and your joints regenerate.

What You'll Need

All you need to do every exercise in this entire book is a sturdy chair, some pillows, and a towel or blanket. That's it.

You may find it helpful to keep a small timer handy. Just set it for five or ten minutes so you won't be distracted looking at the clock. Another option is to undulate to music, which is enjoyable and helps you keep track of time. Of course, you may decide to undulate longer—especially as your body begins to feel better and better.

When to Undulate

One of my favorite times to undulate is right after I wake up. It helps tremendously to soothe away any stiffness that has accumulated in my body while sleeping. You may find that undulation is a wonderful warm up exercise. But if you are one of those who exercise hard, in a way that develops resistance in your body, you would be better served to undulate afterwards, as a gentle cooling down. If you don't currently have a regular exercise program, undulation is ideal. It's invigorating and not difficult, boring, or time-consuming.

You can even sneak undulations into regular daily activities—while in the shower, at the breakfast table, or even in the car waiting at stoplights. It's also the perfect way to unwind, figuratively and literally, at the end of the day.

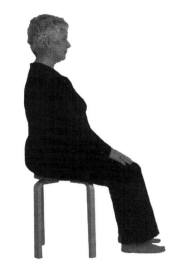

Figure 1.1. Good alignment for sitting

Where to Undulate

Sitting undulations should be done on a firm chair, with both feet firmly on the ground and both sit bones resting evenly on the seat. (See Figure 1.1.) A soft chair or sofa will not provide enough support for your pelvis and jeopardize the alignment to your back and neck. However, an exercise ball is completely acceptable for variation and can be fun and challenging.

Many of the undulations are done on hands and knees. If your knees get sore, simply put a folded towel under them. If getting down onto the floor is difficult, you can use the bed. The mattress surface will not be as beneficial as the floor, but by the very act of undulation, you may soon build enough strength to get there. If your knees are too sore or injured to bear any weight, try hands-and-knees exercises standing with your hands against the wall (as shown in Figure 1.2) and use the wall as you would the floor.

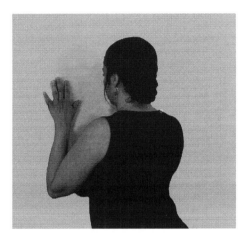

Figure 1.2. If you can't get on your knees, use the wall instead

Also, spread your fingers wide to distribute the weight out over a larger surface area. If your wrists hurt, use fists or elbows and forearms instead. Better yet, alternate between the three positions to strengthen different muscle groups. (See Figure 1.3.)

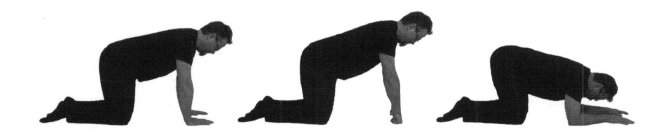

Figure 1.3. Alternate positions when on hands-and-knees to reduce strain on the wrists

It's not a good idea to put anything soft under your wrists or to bend your wrists on a mattress, as that could create strain to the carpal tunnel.

Undulation: Relieve Stiffness and Feel Young

The options of where you can undulate are numerous; anywhere you have the space or inclination. For example, undulating for a minute or two before my chiropractic appointment makes my adjustments smoother. I've even been known to do subtle standing undulations while waiting in line at the grocery store. Not a great suggestion at the bank though; they scrutinize the lines there. Pick a place where you're comfortable and go for it.

How Often and How Much

Practice the Fundamentals every other day, half a minute for each exercise—longer if you can. Do the main undulation at the beginning of the week and then do the variations later in the week. The variations give each undulation a new twist, so to speak.

The amount of time that you practice each day will vary. Three minutes will be enough some days; others you will want to go on for 20 or more. One factor is your condition. Undulation will loosen you up, but occasionally you may find that it's not what your body needs that day. The individual exercise is another factor. When you come across one that is particularly challenging, make an effort to progress, but don't beat yourself up on it. You can't overdo Free Form undulations as long as you breathe, stay aware of your body, avoid painful movements, and stop when you're tired.

Free Form

You will build intelligence into your tissues with this type of exercise. So even though my instructions call for moving a certain way, let your newly astute body take over if there's a different movement that seems necessary at some point. I call this *Free Form*. Free Form will stem from your body's internal knowledge of what's best for it. Anything can be incorporated into your Free Form movements, from earlier undulations to something totally new.

This spontaneity gives your body the opportunity to request what it needs from your movement rather than the typical performance demanded from the body.

Additional Information

Small movements engage your core muscles, those muscles closer to the bones. Large movements engage your sleeve muscles, those closer to the skin. Slow actions initiate from the core moving outward to the sleeve muscles. Fast actions do exactly the opposite, ideally supported by a stable core. When you're unsure if you're engaging the core, simply slow way down. Play with speed and size of different motions to add depth and strength to your muscles.

After a while, you may begin to notice that you usually follow a particular pattern of movement. Once you recognize a pattern, see if you can identify the repetitive movement that could be responsible for it. One example might be to notice that your body twists more easily to the left than to the right. Pay careful attention to the way you get out of your office and/or dining room chair every time. Another may be that you find it difficult to arch your upper back. Is this part of your back slumped in the same position for long periods of time? How many years did it take to develop that pattern? Be patient and reasonable with yourself. You may habitually move at a quick pace. If so, you might truly benefit by slowing down, or vice versa. Your patterns can begin to change the moment you notice them.

Winding Down

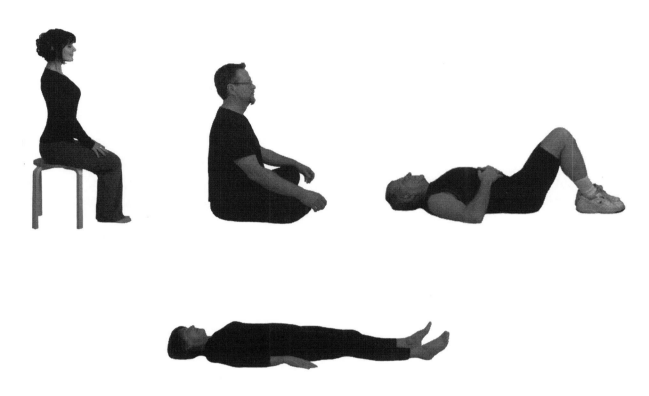

Figure 1.4. Winding down

At the end of each session, rest to let your sensations subside. (Figure 1.4 demonstrates possible resting positions.) This gives your body time to assimilate any changes, and it only takes a moment. If you jump right back into your regular daily routine without this important step, your body reads that as a signal to tighten up and fall back into its same old rut.

Work toward getting a physical sense of your body as water. A fluid state is youthful and strong. Undulations build that flow within—your own internal Fountain of Youth.

What is harder than stone?

What is more soft than water?

Nevertheless hard though rock may be, it is hollowed by the wave.

— Ovid (Publius Ovidius Naso), Roman Poet (First Century BCE)

Notes on the Photographs

The photographs will help people who are visually inclined to get an idea of how each exercise works. Do not feel that you need to copy the model.

The way your body responds to the instructions may be different than what the model's body needed. That's OK. Everyone has unique needs. As long as you listen to your body and try to increase your personal range of motion and ease, you'll be doing the exercises correctly even if your motion does not match the photographs.

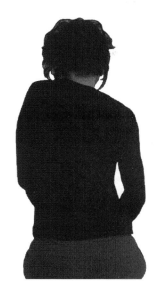

Fundamentals

UNDULATION HAS NO BUILT-IN MEASURE OF ACHIEVEMENT. There's no score or faster time. No perfect pose or weight to add. It's not a competition—even with yourself. If you try to impose a drive for success onto this exercise, you may miss its fundamental benefits.

Consider this: your body knows exactly where it's stuck and what's in its best interests. You don't have to push hard or force beyond its capabilities. Doing what your body wants to do is the grease that lubricates the wheels of fluidity.

Some moves will come easily, others are more challenging. It will always be that way. You may think the goal is to make everything move equally—an impossible task.

The Fundamentals are simple movements (I'm tempted to call them FUNda-mentals) designed to improve your internal observation skills. In addition to waking up your underdeveloped muscles, their focus is to help you learn to listen and see inside your body—where the action is. Let go of the need to achieve and just explore.

Easy Sway

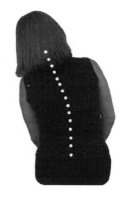 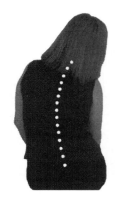 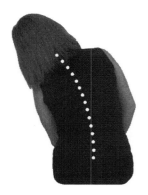

The goal of this exercise is to get to know your spine. Not to be able to move a lot, or to be fluid, but to create fluidity. As you increase your awareness, change will happen naturally. If you currently have back pain, this exercise may offer some relief— a pleasant side effect indeed.

1 Sit in a chair evenly on your sit bones. (Sit on your hands and feel for the hard bumps to find your sit bones. More detailed instructions are in Chapter One. Also, see Figure 1.1.)

2 Move your upper body, swaying from the waist up, to the left and the right.

3 Sway for one minute, noticing which parts of your spine move easily and which are stiff.

4 Stop, breathe, and start again. Initiate a new movement from one of the inflexible places, perhaps from your neck, hips, or between your shoulder blades.

5 As you continue, cast your attention inward to the many different places in your spine. Keep your movements soft and easy.

6 Stop about every minute and begin again from a new place. The quality and quantity of movement will vary depending on what part of your body leads.

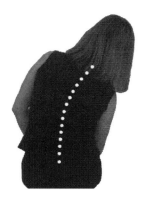 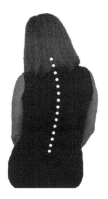 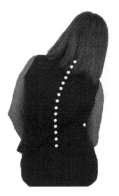

7 Rest for up to one minute or until all of the sensations from your undulations subside.

Variation #1

- ❧ As you sway from side to side, notice the shape of your spine as it curves.

- ❧ First imagine a C-curve with your head and hip on the same side moving toward each other.

- ❧ Move so that the bow or apex of the curve travels up and down your spine. As you do this, the C-curve will temporarily change shape to an S-curve.

- ❧ Let the curve morph from a C-curve to an S-curve and back again over and over.

Variation #2

- ❧ As you sway, notice which parts move a lot, perhaps your neck.

- ❧ Limit the movement of that part so that it moves no more than the places above or below it. Repeat for other over-flexible places.

- ❧ Focus on increasing the movement of stiff places and controlling the movement in over-flexible ones.

However you do this exercise, it is correct.
(The only exception is if you feel pain.)

Reverse the Slouch

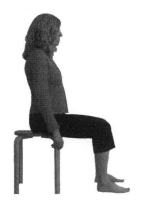 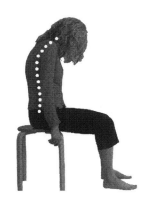 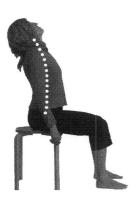

Generally, your spine will probably move more easily in this undulation than in the first exercise. You may find places that are weaker or stickier. Rejoice when you find these blind spots; this is where you can create improved grace.

1   Sit in a chair evenly on your sit bones. It is important for both feet to be firmly planted on the floor.

2   Move your torso so that your sternum dips toward your pelvis and the middle of your back rounds out in back.

3   Move your chest forward and up so that your back arches as the muscles along the sides of your spine contract.

4   Alternate forward and back in this fashion for a minute and notice which parts of your back move easily and which parts don't.

5   Stop about every minute or so and start another movement from a different place. What does it take to get the unyielding places to participate?

6   As you continue, become better acquainted with the front of your spine.

7   Rest for up to a minute, until your back muscles are quiet.

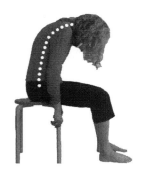 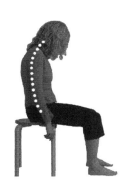 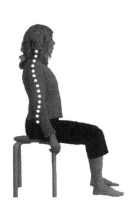

Variation #1

- ❧ Initiate movement from your lower abdominals and pelvis. Pull your pubic bone up toward your chin about an inch.

- ❧ Continue to draw your abdominal muscles in and back so that your chest drops down. Let the movement carry up through your neck so that your chin dips toward your chest.

- ❧ To come back up, start at the base of your spine. Rock your pelvis forward so that your sit bones come back onto the chair surface and your low back returns to its normal curve.

- ❧ Continue the motion flow up from your low back through your middle back, upper back, and through your neck. Straighten your spine until you are sitting tall.

- ❧ Repeat curling in and unfurling, starting both movements from the bottom and working up.

If part of your body doesn't want to move,
breathe into the stuck spot to create an openings

Slo-o-ow Motion

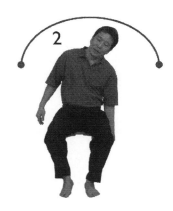 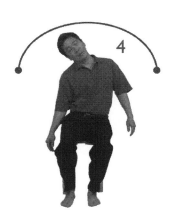 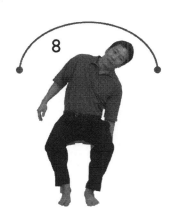

You'll help to develop your intrinsic muscles with this exercise—the muscles most efficient at performing small movements. (I recommend that you listen to music while doing these undulations. Pick a song or two with steady, medium-paced rhythms.)

1   Be seated in a chair on your sit bones, and place both feet firmly on the ground.

2   Begin to undulate in a willowy C-curve, from side-to-side (like Easy Sway), with the music. Listen to the beat and notice the counts used for each undulation. If you're not using music, count out how long it takes for you to get from one side to the other.

3   Sway at this pace for a minute.

4   Now slow down. Double the count it took to complete one revolution. If it took two counts to get from right to left, use four. If it took three, use six, etc.

5   Notice that if parts of the movement feel sticky as you activate the smaller muscles, closer to the core. Undulate side-to-side, at this slower pace, for about a minute or until it becomes easier.

6   Once again, slow down by doubling the count for one revolution. So if your count was four, use eight. Keep your side-to-side C-movement, but notice that the curve may naturally flow into an S-curve in places. Keep breathing, and undulate for a minute at this pace.

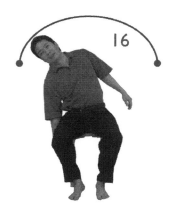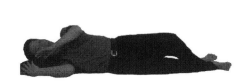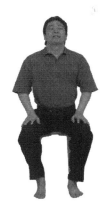

7   You can guess what's coming next, right? Yes, slow down by doubling your count a third time. This would become a count of 16 to undulate from left to right and vice versa. Stay at this pace for a minute or so.

8   If you feel able, slow it down again to a count of 32. Try this for a couple of revolutions.

9   Now let your body choose its own slow pace. It might be a count of 39 or 20 or 15. Do what feels appropriate. When your body finds the rhythm of its core muscles, let loose of the side-to-side movement so that your undulation becomes three dimensional. Stay slow.

10   Sit tall. Reach for the sky with the crown of your head. When you stand up, be aware of how quickly—or slowly—you habitually move.

Variation #1

& Use forward and back movements and repeat the above sequence.

Variation #2

& Undulate slowly in your favorite position: sitting, lying, standing, or on all fours. After a minute or so at that speed, slow down and undulate there for a couple of minutes. Then slow it down again, and again. Find out how slow you can go.

Undulations may feel erratic at first, but they will smooth out as your muscles become hydrated and stronger.

Breathing

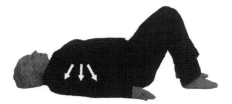 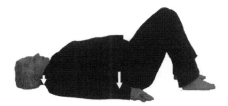

Use undulation to help improve your respiration. Your breath is such a powerful force; it affects all of your organs, energy, and even your mental state. Every cell inside you must breathe to survive.

1   Lie on a hard surface such as the floor with your knees bent and feet flat.

2   Take several breaths. Notice how your chest expands on the inhale relaxes on the exhale.

3   Deepen your breathing and observe how your body moves. Your ribs spread and press into the floor as you inhale.

4   As you exhale, your low back and the back of your neck subtly sink into the floor.

5   Emphasize these movements and imagine yourself floating in the air with each breath in and sinking into the earth as you breathe out.

6   Follow your breath—wherever it takes you—and see what develops. Perhaps it will flow up and down your spine or create a circular movement in your ribs.

7   Rest. Notice if your breath has changed since you began.

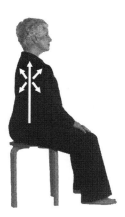 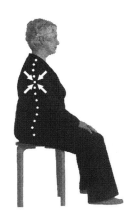

Variation #1

❧ Do this same undulation sitting. On inhale, feel your spine expand and get taller. On exhale, feel your ribs and spine return without collapsing. Enhance and continue.

Variation #2

❧ Lie on your back with your legs straight. Breathe.

❧ Notice how far you can feel breath come into your body. Can you feel subtle a movement in your abdomen? That is your breath wave, caused by your diaphragm pressing against the fluid in your body.

❧ Relax, feel how far out into your arms, legs and head you can ride the wave. Breathe this way for several minutes.

The more you relax, the farther your breath can travel.

Free Form

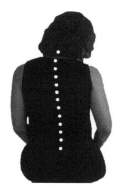 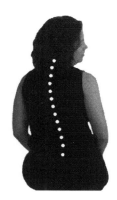 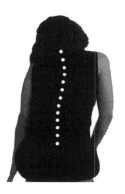

Here's where the magic starts. Your body knows what it needs to be vibrant. If given the opportunity, it will flow into positions your mind couldn't even invent. Listen without judgment or comment. Open the lines of communication and connection to let your body move without restraint.

1. Choose a comfortable position—stand, sit or lie down—and listen to your body for a moment. Breathe.

2. Is there is any place in your body that wants to move? Initiate an undulation from that spot—any way that feels best. Let that movement morph into a different one and then another until it dissipates naturally. If no particular place asks to move, start with one that's stiff or sore.

3. Rest until another place in your body—or maybe the same one again—desires movement. Allow it to move in a way that sparks pleasure. Let this morph into other new movements, until they melt effortlessly away. Rest.

4. Continue letting your undulations arise and subside naturally, until your time is complete.

5. Rest and notice the many, inherent rhythms inside you.

Variation #1

- ❧ Enjoy your favorite undulation for a minute.
- ❧ See if this undulation flows naturally into a different movement.

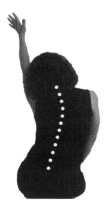 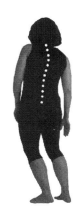 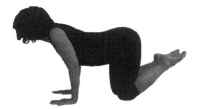

❧ For example, you could start out lying on the floor and pushing through your feet. That could change into a side-to-side rolling, which might easily evolve into being on your hands and knees doing a cat-cow.

❧ I usually start sitting, moving side-to-side, and flow into a spiral/side-to-side/forward-back motion. That move might take me to a standing undulation, with my arms wrapping around and overhead into my own version of modern dance.

Variation #2

❧ Undulate all the way through from standing, to sitting, to lying down, up to hands and knees, back to sitting and finally returning fully upright.

Notice how your mind reacts to
temporarily taking a back seat to your body.

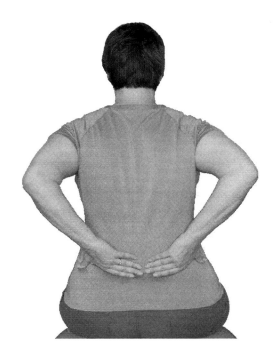

For the Low Back and Hips

DID YOU KNOW THAT BACK PAIN is one of the most common sources of disability? It's a shame that the human back has become so weak and sore in the past 100 years, but not surprising considering how much time we spend in static, uncomfortable positions. Here come undulations to the rescue!

The following five undulations were particularly designed to enliven the muscles and soft tissues of your back and hips. If you've been living with back pain for a while, you might want to go slowly and limit how much you do at first. Don't give up, though. Your back can become strong again, particularly when your hips regain mobility so the spine doesn't have to compensate.

Cat – Cow

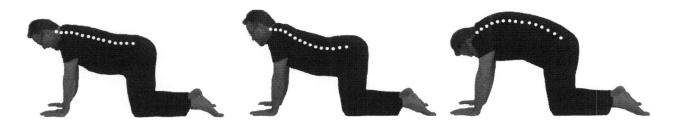

This is a variation of the classic Cat and Cow pose from yoga. It allows your pelvis more freedom to move with the spine. As you rock your pelvis back and forth, how does your low back feel? Awake or tired?

1. Kneel on the floor with your hands shoulder-width apart and knees hip-width apart. If your wrists get sore, interrupt the exercise to take weight off of them for a while. Put a folded towel under your knees if they are tender.

2. As in Reverse the Slouch from the Fundamentals, let your spine move forward (toward the floor) and back (toward the ceiling).

3. Notice how much you use your arms to make your middle back move. Try to let your arms simply hold your upper body weight and let your spine do the work.

4. Continue to move forward and back (also called flexion and extension) and let the movement ripple along your spine from your tailbone to your head and back again.

5. Continue for several minutes. Move slowly at times and quickly at others.

6. Lie down or sit and rest for a minute. Let your body absorb the calm before you hurry off onto your next activity.

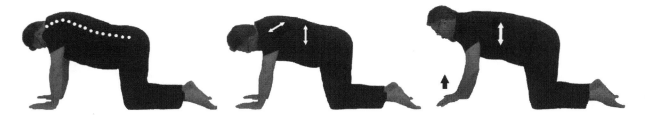

Variation #1

- As you move your spine forward and back, add a little side-to-side movement, which creates a bit of rotation. Like before, notice which parts of your spine resist.

- Stop and let those places decide how to move. The rest of your body will follow.

Variation #2

- As you undulate forward and back, lift one knee slightly to take the weight off of it. Set it back down as you continue to undulate.

- Then lift the opposite hand, just a little bit.

- Continue to undulate, lifting first a knee slightly, then a hand, then the other knee etc. The increased weight on your spine will create new undulation patterns and add strength to the muscles.

If you feel soreness in your low back,
draw your belly button in to support your spine.

Sacrum Stabilizer

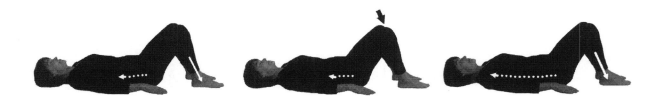

It requires a lot of energy to maintain tension in our bodies. This undulation will help you to release some of that tightness. Rather than force any movement, breathe deeply to help you relax and let go. You will be rewarded with a new sense of ease and comfort.

1   Lie on your back with your knees bent and your feet on the floor. If your chin juts toward the ceiling, fold a small towel and place it under your head to improve the alignment of your neck.

2   In this exercise, it's important to have your hips, knees, and feet aligned. If you keep your knees and feet about four to six inches apart, they will be in line. Try not to let your knees fall in or out.

3   Push your right foot into the floor and feel the force of this travel up your leg and into your pelvis, until it nudges your spine. Release the pressure from your foot.

4   Repeat with your left foot and release; notice how the movement travels differently on this side.

5   Alternate pressing and releasing your feet, with the intention to feel the motion travel up through your torso.

6   When you are relaxed enough, the effect of pushing on your foot will be to move your entire spine. Even your head will move gently to the side.

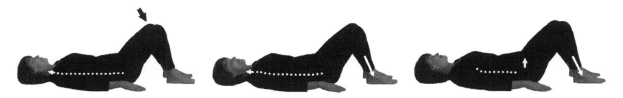

7   The movement will stop in the places where you hold tension. When you notice these points, just be aware of the limitation and encourage more movement.

8   The effect will be different if you use only the ball of your foot or the heel. Try each. Usually it's most effective when you evenly press through your entire foot.

9   Hopefully you feel rested from doing this exercise, but take a minute to check in with your body and release any remaining tension before you get up.

Variation #1

ça Put your arms out to the sides, palms up or down, and create a slight twist with each push.

Variation #2

ça Experiment with the position of your pelvis. Emphasize the curve in your low back, then flatten it, and try to lift your pelvis slightly off the floor.

ça Let your pelvis float into the positions that bring the most movement throughout your spine.

Remember to follow the no-pain guidelines on page 3.

Pelvic Tilt Plus

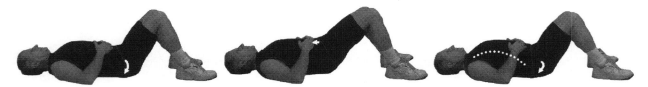

In this undulation—a great spine and hip mobilizer—you'll find building strength can be soothing. Exercise doesn't have to be difficult or cumbersome to be beneficial.

1   Lie on your back with your arms along your sides, and your neck supported if necessary. Bend your knees and keep your feet firmly on the floor to support your body.

2   Press your tailbone to the floor and up towards the back of your head, tilting your pelvis.

3   Feel the arch in your low back and let it continue on up your spine so your middle back, and ribs lift slightly off the floor.

4   Release your pelvis back to neutral. Now bring your pubic bone up toward your chin, tilting your pelvis the other way. Let your low back, middle back, and chest drop into the floor.

5   Continue slowly; for one or two minutes arch your back on your inhale and release it back into the floor on your exhale.

6   Increase the speed of your pelvic tilts; let the movements separate from your breath. You may feel more movement flow through your spine, even though the amount of action in your chest will decrease.

7   Rest if you get tired. When you finish, take a minute to sense the connection between your hips and spine.

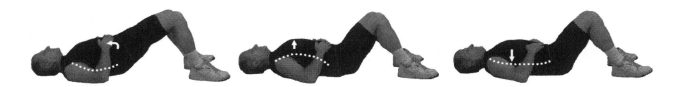

Variation #1

- ❧ Lie as above and lift your chest off the floor and begin the motion from there.

- ❧ Try to use only the muscles around your chest and spine, without help from your shoulders.

- ❧ As you lift your chest, your low back will rise a little and your pelvis may also tilt.

- ❧ Gently release your chest down. Allow your low back to settle into its normal position.

- ❧ Press your chest into the floor so your low back flattens. Follow along with a pelvic tilt.

- ❧ Go slowly at first; lift your chest, then push the back of your ribs into the floor so that the movement flows through your entire back.

- ❧ Vary the speed of your movements.

Use your abdominal muscles to pull your pelvis up
rather than pushing with your buttocks.

Happy Dog

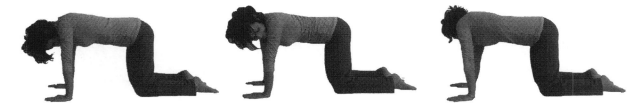

Up Dog and Down Dog are common yoga postures. Here is a variation developed by one of my lovely clients, Nancy Logan, during her daily exercise routine. I call it Happy Dog, because it always puts me in a good mood.

1   Get on your hands and knees. Place your hands directly under your shoulders and your knees directly under your hip joints. See Figure 1.3 on page 6 for variations that are easy on your wrists.

2   Look under your left shoulder at your left knee. Now look past the outside of your arm at your left foot.

3   Come back to the starting position, looking straight down at the floor. Then repeat the sequence on your right side.

4   Inhale as you come back to neutral and exhale as you twist.

5   As you continue to alternate from side-to-side, notice how much movement is happening in your neck and how much in the rest of your spine. Take a deep breath and direct both the inhale and exhale down your spine to unlock any bracing.

6   Look at your knees and feet again. Slowly wind and unwind, letting the movement that starts in your neck travel all the way down to your tailbone. Continue for several minutes alternating sides.

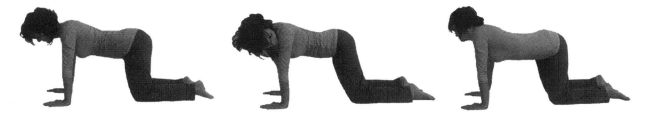

7   Release the movement of your spine. Let your undulations migrate freely and follow the whims of your body. Undulate this way for several more minutes.

8   Sit and relax until all the sensations ebb from your body; keep the newfound freedom in your neck and hips.

Variation #1

- ❧ Do the undulation as above, but look over your shoulders to your derriere.

- ❧ Follow the entire motion with your eyes.

Variation #2

- ❧ On your hands and knees as above, bring your tailbone toward the crown of your head on the right. Then go to the left.

- ❧ Experiment. First have the movement start from your tail and extend up to your head, and then opposite; start with your neck and flow down your spine. Try to feel the movement occur in all parts of your spine simultaneously and evenly.

Look only as far as you can without causing pain even if that means you can't see your foot or rear end.

Hip Hiker

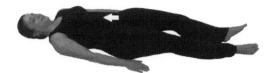 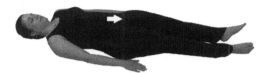

Back pain is often associated with weak, tight hips. This undulation will strengthen, release and massage those overloaded muscles in your low back and hips.

1   Lie on your back, on the floor, legs straight. If you need extra support for your low back, put pillows lengthwise under your legs.

2   Slowly wiggle your hips. Notice what you feel there and in your low back.

3   Keep your buttocks on the floor and draw your left hip up towards your left armpit, but not toward the ceiling. Hold for a count of three then release it back down to the start position. Repeat on the right side.

4   Do the movement again, but slower. Take a full count of five to hike your hip and another five to return. As you move, notice what happens in your low back and how far up your spine you can feel the undulation. Repeat on the right.

5   Make the movements bigger if you can; play with smaller ones.

6   Now you can let your buttocks lift off the ground as you move. Try not to over-stretch; remember, let your sensations guide you.

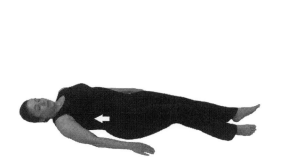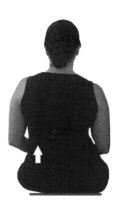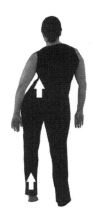

7   Continue for several minutes; alternate sides and speeds. See what causes the movement to travel up your body the farthest.

8   Let the movement from your hips and low back travel through—and engage—the rest of your body.

9   Lie still for a moment. Notice how your hips and low back feel. Get up carefully; your low back had a good workout.

Variation #1

& Do the same undulation sitting on a firm chair or exercise ball. As you lift each hip to your armpit, let your weight shift in opposition, from sit bone to sit bone.

Variation #2

& Do the undulation standing up.

Remain conscious of your pain signals. (Are you getting a yellow caution light, a red stop light, or are the lights all green?)

Undulation: Relieve Stiffness and Feel Young

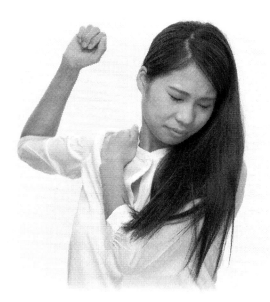

For Neck, Shoulders, & Arms

The proverbial pain in the neck seems to be getting more widespread nowadays. Perhaps it's due to the time spent on our electronic devices or lack of movement in general. Often, neck pain is the result of lack of range of motion in the shoulders – and shoulder and arm pain can be a result of restrictions in the neck. That's why the undulations in this section address the three together.

Snake Arms

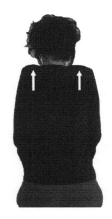 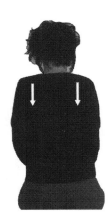 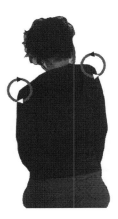

My office is full of clients with back pain caused by their backs doing the work of their shoulders and vice versa. They are ecstatic when I release the connective tissue that binds their shoulder blades and ribs. Freedom! This exercise is a self-massage that will release your shoulders and back.

Sit down or stand up.

1. Lift your shoulders up toward your ears and hold for a couple of seconds. Then let them drop. Repeat this a few times.

2. Next lift your shoulders slightly, release and pull them down toward your hips and hold a couple of seconds. Repeat this several times.

3. Undulate your shoulders in circles, forward, up, over, and back — together and then alternate.

4. Notice if your back is moving with your shoulders. Move them independently as much as you are able.

5. Next, undulate your torso forward-and-back and side-to-side without lifting your shoulders or drawing them forward.

6. Initiate your movements from your spine and let them flow out through your arms, elbows, wrists, and fingers.

7. After several minutes, reverse and let your arms lead your body into new undulations. Add movement where ever it feels appropriate.

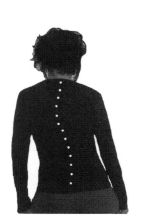 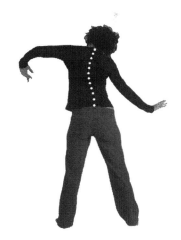 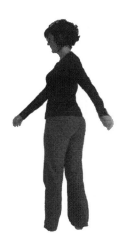

8 Bring stillness into your body. Rest until all sensation subsides.

Variation #1

- Stand with your feet comfortably apart and flexible knees.
- Lean to one side. As you lean, reach your arm out to that same side.
- Come back to center. Move from your spine first; draw your body toward the opposite side and reach with the other arm.
- This is a form of "snake arms" from belly dance. Let your spine and shoulders roll with the movements, all the way through your neck and out the top of your head.
- Be careful of whiplash with your neck. As you get more comfortable with this movement, spread your feet farther apart so that your body can sway further to each side.

Variation #2

- Stand with your arms at your sides. Twist your torso from side to side and let your arms swing around with you.
- If your arms are flying free, they will flap your front and backside.
- Continue for two minutes, then let your movement digress from rotation to side bending and back again, letting your arms follow the movements of your torso.

Let your shoulder blades slide around
on your ribs and your arms be free.

Octopus

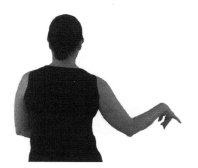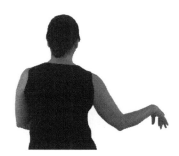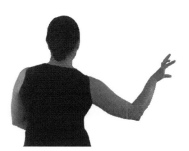

Stiff joints are the bane of the elderly and usually the first symptom people associate with feeling their age. Kim Illig taught me this exercise to soothe my hands after I became a Hellerwork practitioner. It worked wonders for my sore fingers. My clients with arthritis also report its benefits.

This exercise can be done in any position.

1   Curl and unfurl the fingers and thumb of the hand that you use most often. Imagine you are an octopus waking up the ends of your tentacles.

2   For a minute or so, see how fluid your fingers can become. Flush out the inflexibility from your knuckles.

3   Let the movement creep up your hand to incorporate the wrist.

4   Continue the flow up the arm to include the elbow and then the shoulder.

5   Let the movement from your fingers, wrist, elbow, and shoulder influence the rest of your body for a minute.

6   Repeat the sequence with your other hand.

7   Now move both hands and arms. Imagine an octopus swimming in the ocean.

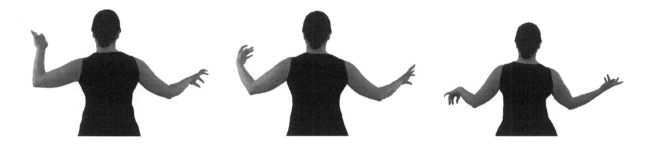

8   Involve your entire body and evolve into a Free Form undulation.

9   Sit or lie with your hands in your lap. Feel softness and lightness in your joints.

Variation #1

&   Change your position. For example, if you were sitting, stand this time or lie down.

As you try new movements, you may not feel fluid at first.
That will change with practice.

Yes-No-Maybe So

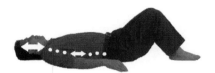 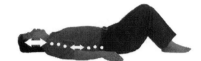 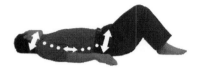

Simple, everyday movements can turn into organic, productive undulations. Involve more of your body and add a twist to the ordinary, as in this exercise where a firm nod of the head wobbles down to pliable hips.

1   Lie flat on your back.

2   Nod your head "yes" repeatedly. Include your neck and back in the movement—all the way down to your tailbone.

3   Shake your head "no." Swivel through your body so your shoulders and pelvis rock.

4   Merge "yes" and "no" into a topsy-turvy motion that engages the rest of your body.

5   Do all of the above, but start from your hips with up-down (yes), side-to-side (no) and all around (maybe so). Carry the movement up through your spine and skull.

6   Maybe So is a type of Free Form in itself. Take your already loose undulations off the floor into a crawling or standing Free Form.

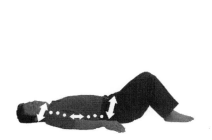 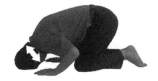 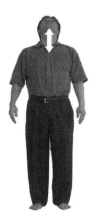

7 Rest for a minute. You don't necessarily have to be still to do so.

Variation #1

    ❧ Kneel with your forehead on the floor and repeat the above sequence.

Variation #2

    ❧ Do it all standing.

Paint Your Head with the Floor

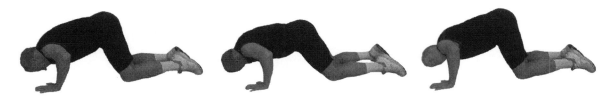

This exercise is great for a stiff neck. It originated with Contact Improvisation, a playful, spontaneous dance form. I learned it from Stuart Bell and Gita Sivander.

1 Start on your hands and knees with your forehead on the ground.

2 Gently rock your forehead so that each part of it touches the floor.

3 Move so all the different parts of your face come into contact with the floor. Notice what little, unusual movements are necessary to get all around your nose and chin.

4 The fun part is to get every part of your scalp to touch, especially around your ears. To touch your entire head to the floor, you'll need to roll onto your side and then your back.

5 Don't force any movements! Let your neck unwind at its own pace, so your skull swivels on top of your vertebrae. Give it the necessary time.

6 Stuart explained the exercise like this: pretend the floor is covered in wet paint; to transfer the paint to your body (in this case your head) you need to make direct contact.

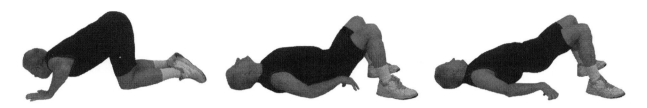

7   Continue "painting" down your body.

8   Shake like a wet dog to get all the paint off yourself.

9   Rest, very aware of your skin.

Variation #1

- ∂ Lie on your back, legs bent and feet on the ground. Start the undulation with the back of your head rolling on the floor.

- ∂ Paint as far up your skull as you can. Try to get all of the nooks and crannies around the ears.

- ∂ Now roll over to your forehead and face. This reverses the order so you start on your back and finish on your hands and knees or side.

People often restrain movements to avoid looking odd or different.
Imagine how much vitality they lose to stay "normal."

Neck Detangler

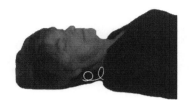 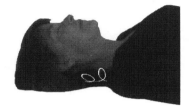 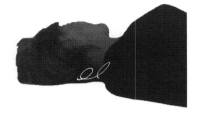

This exercise is intended to help unlock stiffness in your neck. Overloaded and cramped muscles can cause the connective tissue around them to get tangled, like a length of rope that has been jumbled in a bag. If you pull hard on a tangle, it only tightens the knots. In order to loosen them, it's necessary to create slack.

1. Lie on your back with your legs in any position that is comfortable for your low back.

2. Visualize the vertebrae in your neck. (See the drawings on page 91.) The spinous process that poke out the back, the transverse processes that stick out each side, and the front of each vertebra in the center of your neck.

3. Imagine a long string that wraps all around your neck bones.

4. Wobble your head and sway your neck to search out and detangle— as gently as you would a delicate gold chain—a tangled, sore spot in your neck.

5. Unwind away from that spot with side to side and circling motions.

6. As one spot lets go, another may pop up with symptoms. Loosen each tight spot that you feel.

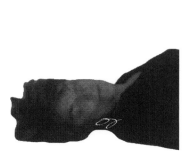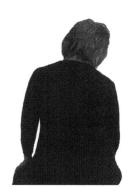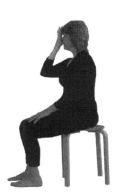

7   Continue unraveling down your spine. Engulf your whole body in a Free Form undulation.

8   Rest and be aware of your entire neck; include your throat, the spaces under your ears, and in between all the vertebrae.

Variation #1

- Sit in a chair to do this exercise.

- The muscles in your neck will have to work differently to support the weight of your head.

- This position also gives you the ability to tilt your head back as you unwind.

Variation #2

Create *Nose Circles* as follows:

- Put your palm flat against your nose.

- Draw a circle with your nose on your hand. Make it as smooth and round as you can.

- Go the other way.

- Spiral in and out.

- Try your other hand.

If your pain could express itself in words,
what would it say?

Undulation: Relieve Stiffness and Feel Young

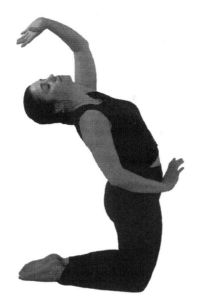

Chapter Two

The Fountain of Youth

IN THE VERY BEGINNING OF OUR LIVES, all we did was undulate. We began undulating in the womb; the motion carried us into this world. We undulated and wiggled in our cribs. Those first attempts to crawl were simply ingenious versions of undulation. Through standing and early walking we remained fluid, but then the bigger world of school and work required conformity. Our agility decreased, consistent with society's demands for stillness and repetitive motion. It's not a lost cause though; anyone can regain some of what was left behind in those early years.

To Counteract Aging

Loss of mobility, arthritis, and frailty are often considered natural and unavoidable parts of aging, but unlike many people assume, they are not fait accompli. It's true, however, that some of our misconceptions about wellness—no pain without gain and if a little of something is good, then a lot of it is better—lead to that end. To stay nimble, it's important to work smarter, not harder. Joints that are used in their full range of motion are less likely to get arthritis. Increasing flexibility little by little is vastly more effective that trying to get it in one big stretch. These undulations are designed to keep you mobile, and they are fun, an important ingredient of youthful activity.

My Encounters with Undulation

Growing up, I embraced the world that rejected the body's need to move. I was blessedly thin, and to "look good" I didn't feel the need to exercise, so my core strength didn't develop. Since my self worth depended mainly on mental accomplishments, I didn't identify with my body at all. What's more, I thought that my brain deserved a way better body as a container and would have traded for a curvier, coordinated, athletic one if given half a chance.

That all worked pretty well; until I was in my 30s that is. Suddenly mysterious aches and pains appeared as my body wore out. Confidence in my body's ability to meet my brain's demands evaporated. It should not have come as any surprise—but it did. I had been making continual withdrawals from my physical bank account after all, living off the interest and depleting principal generated by childhood activity.

I might have accepted the fate of general physical decline—millions of us do—if I hadn't found Hellerwork Structural Integration.[1] I was fortunate.

My Hellerwork practitioner rebalanced my soft tissue, taught me how maintain good alignment . . . and to undulate. Undulation is the classic movement lesson given during the sixth session of the Hellerwork Series.

I was frustrated when I tried to mimic an illustration in The Hellerwork Client Handbook. It showed a model demonstrating a beautiful, even, flowing, side-to-side undulation. (See Figure 2.1.) I couldn't get my body to move like that.

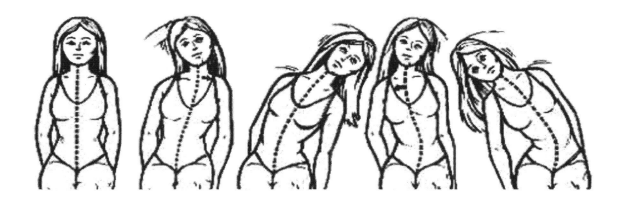

Figure 2.1. Undulation (Reprinted from the Hellerwork Client Handbook with kind permission from Hellerwork International, LLC.)

A revolution in my life came during an assignment during my training to become a Hellerwork practitioner. We undulated every day for a week. I was still disappointed by my imperfections, but after several days I noticed my movements were much easier

---

[1] Hellerwork Structural Integration is holistic modality that helps people return to a more balanced, aligned and fluid state. It combines deep-tissue bodywork with movement education and awareness dialogue in a series of eleven sessions.

and flowing more like the picture! Just those five minutes of undulation every day produced excellent results and helped my back feel so much better. And I began to undulate almost every day.

With this new found freedom of movement, I felt confident enough to try activities I never dreamed I could do, including yoga and belly dance. Many yoga postures move the spine between flexion (curved forward) and extension (arched into a small backbend). The style of yoga I selected, Viniyoga, includes a pose that emphasized a flow between stretching the chest and low back. (See Figure 2.2) In Belly dance there are many figure-8 movements and combinations of the hips, arms and spine. (Figure 2.3 is a photo of my lovely belly dance teacher, Aleili.) The best belly dancers can combine many layers of undulations at once. I added new movements from both these ancient art forms to my growing repertoire.

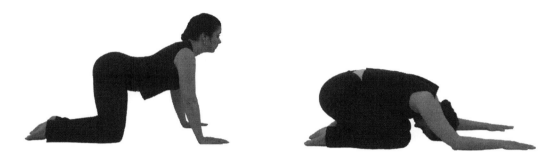

Figure 2.2. Viniyoga pose, Chakravakasana, which flows between stretching the front of the spine and the back.

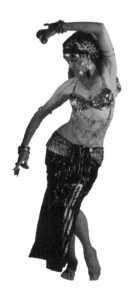

Figure 2.3. My beautiful teacher, Aleili. (Reprinted with kind permission of Aleili.)

During this time, I had the honor to meet and take a workshop from Emilie Conrad, the founder of Continuum Movement. Emilie moves with as much grace and strength as anyone I have ever seen—and she is over 70 years old! Many consider her to be the

Queen of Undulation. (See Figure 2.4 for a photo of beautiful and dynamic Emilie.) She certainly proved to me that the breakdown we call getting old can be stalled by frequently accessing our internal flow.

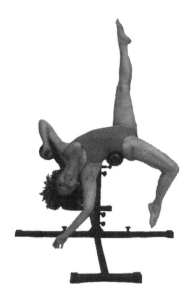

Figure 2.4. Emilie Conrad, founder of Continuum Movement, Inc. (Reprinted with kind permission of Continuum Movement.)

Undulations are Natural

By the time we become adults, most of us have been disconnected from our bodies for so long, we can't remember it any other way. If we could remember the mind-body bond, we'd realize that many of our fundamental processes depend on undulation—like the feeling of our hearts beating, the whisper of our breath, or the gurgles of normal digestion. In addition, more subtle waves exist in the lymph system, craniosacral rhythm, and visceral patterns.

What we commonly think of as aging is disruption in the flow of these systems. Joseph Heller, the founder of Hellerwork Structural Integration, and William Henkin describe it well in *Bodywise:*

> "The process of life may be seen as one in which we start out 99% water and end up virtually solid… In the course of aging, most of us find ourselves increasingly sedentary and confined, moving less and less. We may claim our static state results from pain, fatigue or laziness, but which, in fact, comes first? To function properly, the body relies heavily on the movement of fluids, and as rigidity sets in the fluid flow is impaired."

Life depends on layers of rhythms: fluids that pulse under pressure and others that seep, vibrations of sound and brain waves. All are undulations. By incorrectly assuming the body is a combination of levers and pulleys—with off and on switches to operate them—we limit the variety of our movements, as though we were a part of an assembly line. This abuse is partially responsible for the abundance of repetitive strain injuries and arthritis in our society.

Childhood – Playful Pursuits

Toddlers are able to move in a variety of directions with ease and simple pleasure. You did too when you were a child. Cast your mind back to all the wonderful things that you could do when you were little, many of which are now rare and some of which you might not have done in years.

Dance	Sit on the floor
Squat	Jump
Kick your legs	Walk on your toes
Shake your hips	Run
Reach way up high	Skip
Twirl around	Climb a tree
Swing	Jump rope
Crawl more than five feet	Put your foot in your mouth (literally)

When my children were small, I spent more time at the park. I noticed that two and three year-olds stood up like they were sprouting from the earth—exactly how I try to teach my clients to stand. The kids were a little wobbly when learning to walk, but that smoothed out beautifully after a year or so.

Four-year olds had the grace of adults and the vitality of toddlers.

But around age five or six those same children began to stiffen. Does aging really start to happen that young? Well, yes and no. The body is fully capable of retaining its fluid nature, but it gets short-circuited as we are required to sit still for longer and longer periods each day. Except for short bursts during recess, that endless variety of activity gets lost, starting with school.

Adolescents – Socialized and Conditioned

When we adapt to a group setting, self-centered individuality is traded for self-conscious conformity. Avoiding ridicule often limits outward self-expression and likewise restricts movement. In addition, girls may slouch to hide a maturing bosom—a posture that further diminishes physical connection.

For another example, look at the way people walk. Even though a healthy pelvis has the ability to move in three dimensions, (as shown in Figure 2.5) many adults hold their pelvis still when they walk. Why? Because our society has deemed that certain motions are considered taboo for women and especially for men. We've been taught that allowing our hips their full range of motion, even in a normal walking pattern, is too sexy or effeminate. It's really too bad, because hips only gain flexibility and strength when simply allowed to swivel and sway with every step.

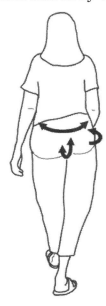

Figure 2.5 Healthy walking doesn't limit natural movement of the hips.

Adulthood – The Machine

If a child skipped from the car to the grocery store, we would think nothing of it and might even be amused by it. But why is it odd when an adult skips? A successful adult is enmeshed in the gears of modern life; wound up to work with precision and not stray from the path of expectation. Adulthood includes being level-headed, braced to handle any circumstance, and carrying the weight of responsibility firmly on one's shoulders—all forms of stiffness. The very idea of how an adult *should* act accentuates existing restrictions—a primary factor in getting old.

The conditions that we normally associate with aging—stiffness of the joints, arthritis, osteoporosis, hardening of the arteries, the drain of energy, loss of strength, and those all-over general aches and pains—are completely opposite of the soft and supple conditions we associate with youth.

In this era of disposable everything, many expect the body to wear out and fail, like a car or coffee maker. And like mechanical objects that deteriorate without care, so too will our bodies if we neglect regular maintenance. Lavish the care on yourself that you would a fine Rolls Royce. After all, your body is more valuable than any car.

However, unlike machines, our bodies are actually living organisms, which give us the amazing ability to heal and regenerate. But since all our repair and immune system cells need to flow through the connective tissue to get to all areas of the body, healing is a fluid process.

The Aged – Paying the High Price

The conveniences of the modern world save us time and effort, but they also erode the breadth of our movement and core strength. It's hard to stay still when gardening or listening to music on the radio. By contrast, watching TV generally produces a state of inactivity that borders on comatose. People also tend to accommodate decreasing range of motion. They install higher toilet seats and stop putting items on the top shelf. Many believe that every decade older entitles one to do less with the body. Unfortunately the gradual reduction of activity can leave you confined to chair or bed. (See Figure 2.6.)

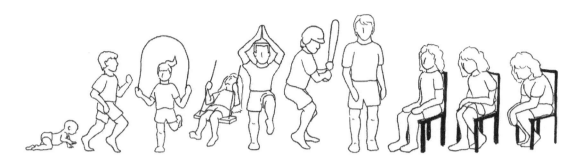

Figure 2.6 The cycle of life can be seen as increasing and then decreasing activity.
Illustration by Dana Young.

If we look around us, we can see varying degrees of degeneration even among people of the same age. For instance, over a million and a quarter adults age 75 and older were residents in a nursing home in 1999. And yet other seniors are still full of life, able to spring up in the morning and go strong throughout the day. The International Health, Racquet and Sportsclub Association reports that 25% of their 41.3 million members are over the age of 55.

Did you know that there are even seniors who are elite athletes? More than 180 people, aged 70 and older, completed the Boston Marathon in 2016. Wow!

How is it possible that some 74-year-olds hobble to the bathroom, while others run marathons? While genetics and luck play a part in the aging process, I'll show you that how you move your body is also a huge factor. If most of us start feeling some stiffness and inflexibility as early as age 30, is it truly possible to remain fluid and healthy? Definitely! I'll get you started on your way with the low-impact exercises in this book. Best of all? A marathon is not required.

Getting it Back

I've seen many people, of many different ages, recover from stillness-induced dysfunction. Structural Integration, physical therapy, yoga, Pilates, circuit training, regular walking, and other modalities can be effective, because every system in your body depends on physical activity for good health. Undulation is an essential ingredient in all these therapies, even though it's not usually thought of separately.

To supplement the movement education I offer as a Hellerwork practitioner, I've hosted a number of undulation workshops for my clients. They loved the freedom undulation gave them and how it helped relieve their aches and pains. My clients noticed how this movement had a dual character: simple, but not always easy; odd, but somehow familiar; amazingly effective, but without the extra effort that most felt necessary to produce results.

The Fountain of Youth

The flow generated from inside the body creates amazing strength and flexibility, and it's best accessed when you can let go of the need to consciously control movement. Part way through an undulation, you'll suddenly become aware of just where your body is, and think "Wow, I wouldn't have believed I could do this!"

Undulation enables you to move better and when done regularly, you may start to notice that other forms of exercise like golf, swimming, walking, tennis, or dance begin to get easier; because a fluid body is capable of moving in any direction, as well as being equally both strong and flexible.

My clients' success and enthusiasm motivated me to write this book. While some of my clients took to undulation like fish to water, most preferred to have instructions. During my daily undulations, I regularly found something new that I wanted to teach others. This book contains only 48 of the exercises from my discoveries plus variations.

You'll find that the potential of your body is truly unlimited, though it might not feel like that now. This book will walk you through many simple but uncommon movements and will help you gradually improve the condition of your joints and muscles. Soon, you'll be reconnected to the fluid nature of yourself. Don't be surprised when you feel younger. Undulation can generate a deep well of fluid flooding up your spine and spreading out through your connective tissue. This is the Fountain of Youth that *you* can discover.

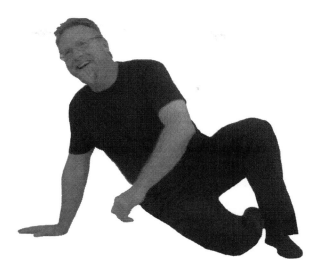

To Counteract Aging

To grow in age is desirable and inevitable. To become decrepit and feeble is not. While the course we take as we get older is somewhat determined by fate, we have control over a large portion of our destiny. Stiffness—even for those who have arthritis—can be diminished. Strength can be maintained, although it does require more dedicated effort. To feel younger, we need to move like we did when we were children. The following undulation exercises are designed to recreate the awareness, fluidity, and playfulness of youth.

Feel Your Spine

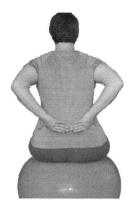 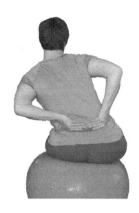 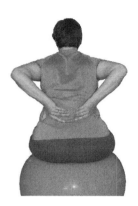

In this exercise, you touch your vertebrae to stimulate movement. Tactile input enriches awareness and mobility, and also helps you identify where you are actually stuck. Interestingly enough, this is usually not where it hurts. Normally, you'll find limited movement just above or just below the painful spots.

1   Sit in a chair with both feet on the floor.

2   Put your hands at the base of your low back over your hip bones with your thumbs facing forward and fingers on your sacrum, as shown in the first photo. Your sacrum is the large bone at the base of your spine that rests in between your pelvis bones, connecting at the notorious sacro-iliac joints.

3   Rock your sacrum around—forward-back, side-to-side, rotation—and notice what small movements happen easily.

4   Slide your fingers up a bit to feel for a bony prominence, an inch or so below the level of your hip bones. This is the spinous process of your lumbar vertebra. Now, move from this point and notice which movements come easily.

5   Find the next bone up and repeat the process. A light touch typically works better than pressing hard.

6   Change the position of your hands to counteract any strain in your arms or fingers. Continue all the way up your spine. You'll need to reach over your shoulder at some point to get the places in your upper back.

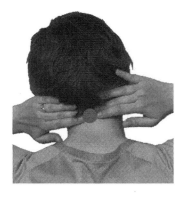 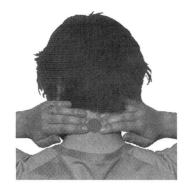 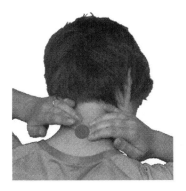

7 You cannot feel the bone in an area, try moving your body so that you can feel it indirectly. Not all spinous processes are close to the skin, especially if you have extra tight muscles or a vertebra out of alignment.

8 Include movements from each of the seven vertebrae in your neck. You will not be able to feel the upper most vertebrae, but use the back of your skull as a substitute

9 Once you reach the top, wiggle and squirm to involve every vertebra in order from top to bottom.

10 Rest, sitting or lying down, until your back is at peace.

Variation #1

☙ The variation for this exercise is simply to notice the difference in your movement from day to day.

Variation #2

☙ You can also ask someone to touch your vertebrae for you.

*The good news is that the more often you do this exercise,
the more flexible your arms, shoulders, and back will become.*

Walking

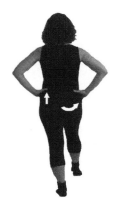 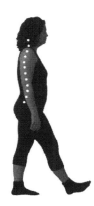 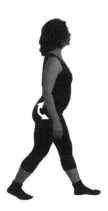

Walking is the ultimate human exercise. Simultaneously energizing and relaxing, it can stimulate your entire body with undulations that naturally flow and merge from one into another.

1   Find an area where you can walk for ten or more paces, perhaps around your living room, down a long hallway, or outside.

2   Put your hands on your hips and walk. Notice how your pelvis tilts and swivels.

3   As your weight transfers from one leg to the other, each hand will rise higher and forward of the other with the motion of the hip. Release unnecessary tension in your hips and low back to encourage the motion.

4   Let your hands fall naturally to your sides. Keep walking and notice how your spine can undulate as the pelvis moves.

5   Your shoulders will naturally follow the movement of everything below them and they'll glide with each step, unless your muscles are grabbing and holding on to prevent it. Do your shoulders glide?

6   Walk for a minute with the intention of allowing your torso, shoulders, arms, and hands to all follow your hips.

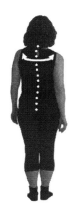 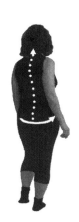 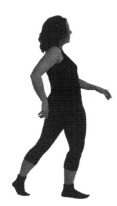

7   As your spine undulates, your head may want to nod a bit. Let it wobble.

8   walk and sense the movement coming up from your feet, into the pelvis, through the spine, and out the top of your head.

9   When you are finished walking, sit for a minute. Notice how your head and feet—and everything in between—feel connected.

Variation #1

ও Walk and exaggerate all of the above movements: hips swaying, arms swinging, and head nodding.

When you incorporate undulation into your daily activities
the benefits increase exponentially.

Crawling

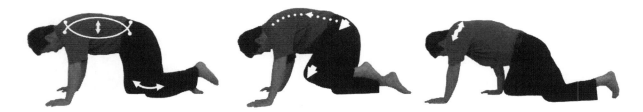

One way to recover a youthful feeling in your body is to recreate a childhood movement, such as crawling. You'll find several, synchronized undulations in this exercise.

1   Get on your hands and knees.

2   Lift one knee slightly. Swing it back and forth so your back sways and arches. Feel the effect up to your neck. (The first undulation.)

3   Bring the knee forward and put weight on it; feel your sacrum and low back shift over to that side only about an inch or two. When you push through your knee, lower leg and the top of the foot, your spine will be propelled forward in a wave. (The second undulation.)

4   When the wave reaches your upper back, reach the opposite arm forward.

5   Transfer the weight over to this arm from the other one and consciously generate a purposeful undulation from shoulder to shoulder. (The third undulation.)

6   Focus on the trio of undulations as you crawl slowly.

7   Release your concentration and crawl at a comfortable pace.

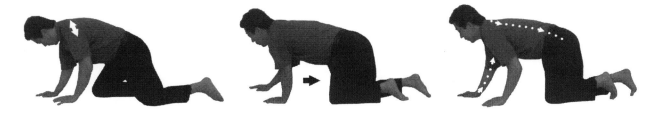

8   Move to a Free Form undulation on hands and knees and then other positions.

9   As you rest, invite the playfluness of yourself as a two-year-old to stay.

Variation #1

- ❧ Crawl backwards.

- ❧ As you push from your hand, feel the motion travel through your arm, shoulder, and spine to the opposite hip.

- ❧ Create a slight arch in your spine with the intention to feel each vertebra articulate.

Remember to breathe through your body
to enhance your undulations.

Follow the Music

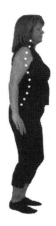 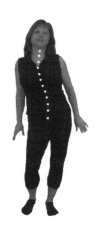 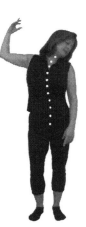

Music speaks to us deeply. Do you have songs that you love? Let your body express your favorite music so you can enjoy it physically as well as mentally.

Put on a song that moves your spirit. It doesn't matter what type of music it is: classical, rock, country, or swing—any kind will work. Choose something five to ten minutes long.

1   Pretend the instruments are inside you and your body is playing the music.

2   Physically respond to the notes. Let how you feel show through your face, arms, legs, and spine.

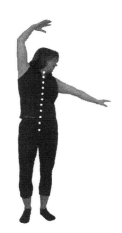 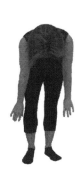 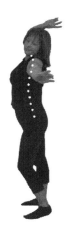

3 Suspend judgment about how you look. There's no right or wrong way to dance. It only has to feel good.

4 Rest for a minute. Take as much pleasure in your body as you do the music.

Variation #1

ॐ Use different music.

Creativity is a natural, fluid process.

Tailbone Penmanship

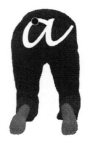 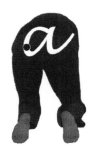 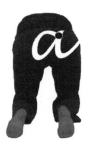

Low back muscles commonly over-stabilize the spine and become stiff. It's difficult to move when the lumbar vertebrae are mortared together like concrete blocks. This undulation softens the mortar and mobilizes the blocks.

1 Get on your hands and knees, with your hands directly under your shoulders and your knees directly under your hip joints.

2 Warm up your body for a minute. Move your hips, back, and shoulders.

3 Pretend your tailbone is a laser pointer that sends a beam of red light to the floor between your ankles.

4 Draw a cursive letter "a" with your laser pointer. Take your time and try to smooth out the curves.

5 Go through the alphabet from "a" to "z." Try to initiate most of the movement from your pelvis, rather than your legs, so your hips swivel on your thigh bones and nudge your spine from side to side.

6 Coordinate the movement of your tail and spine to create more flexibility in your low back.

7 Write your name.

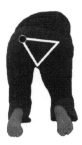 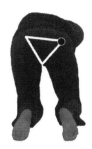 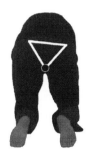

8   Write the alphabet again in upper case letters, if you feel like your body
    wants to continue.

9   Lie on your back. Feel the swimming feeling in your low back. Disperse
    the sensation throughout your body and move into Free Form.

10 Bring your movement to a close and rest.

Variation #1

☙ Draw shapes instead of letters: circles, triangles, stars, clouds, zigzags, and
  spirals. Anything you can think of.

Variation #2

☙ Draw each letter slowly. Take 10 seconds for each one.

Feel your confidence grow each time you try something new.

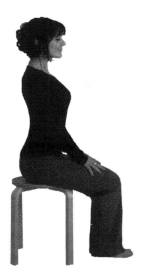

For Better Posture

Here's a chicken and an egg question for you: What came first, bad posture or bad movement? It doesn't matter what comes first; they go together and compound each other. Conversely, improving your posture will result in better movement. These exercises are much more effective, sustainable, and fun than pulling your shoulders back.

Fountain

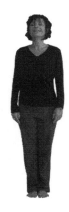 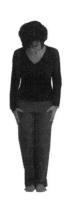 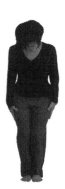

You are creating your own Fountain of Youth as you go through the undulations in this book. This exercise is a physical metaphor of your body regaining its vitality. If your idea of the fountain is different than mine, go with your image, not the instructions I've listed below.

1   Stand with your feet close together.

2   Imagine you're on top of a geyser and water gurgles under your feet. Feel the water spread beneath your arches, surge up your legs, into your torso, and spray from the crown of your head.

3   Press your feet into the ground. Lift your upper body and grow to your full height.

4   Imagine ebb in the flow. Relax, without collapsing, back down. Bend your knees. Feel the imaginary water drain down the inside of your body, into an underground river, and transport all the stress and toxins with it as it goes.

5   When the geyser erupts again, activate your core and expand from the inside out.

6   As the surge subsides, let yourself curl inward.

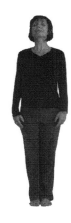 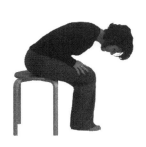 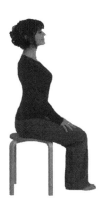

7   Spout upwards again.

8   After you complete several ebbs and flows, walk like you are a water fountain.

9   Turn this into a Free Form undulation.

10   Rest in any position. Notice the fluids inside you.

Variation #1

   ❧ Sit and go through the undulation. With your legs taken out of play, your core muscles will really get involved.

Your body is more than 50% water. Can you feel it?

Balance Scale

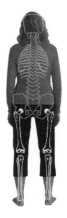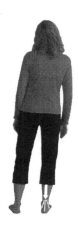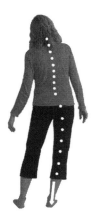

This exercise builds balance. Maintaining your equilibrium requires flexibility and strength—and the adaptability to counter the uneven inevitabilities of life.

1   Stand with your feet hip width apart and knees flexible. If you need support, stand next to a wall or table.

2   Feel the floor under your feet. Trust your feet and legs to hold you up. How often do they let you down, after all?

3   Consciously relax your rigid muscles. Allow your bones to float within your body—and your balance to shift from one leg to the other.

4   Counterbalance with your upper body in response to the fluctuating base of support.

5   Emphasize the transfer of weight from one foot to the other. Experiment putting the weight on different parts of your feet: heels, balls, inside, and outside.

6   Continue this cycle: shift weight → upper body responds → lower body shifts in response to upper body → upper body responds, etc.

7   Let your movements grow as you become more comfortable. How far can you sway and still maintain a confident balance?

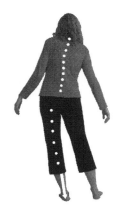 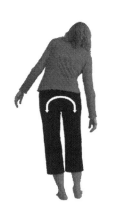 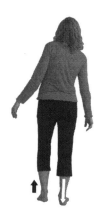

8   Slowly shift the weight of your hips around. Include your arms.

9   Move into a Free Form undulation. Follow your body's desires.

10   Rest. Notice your body wants to stay upright automatically; it doesn't require tension.

Variation #1

❧ Increase and decrease the space between your feet. Notice the different muscles in play when your feet are close together or farther apart.

Variation #2

❧ Lift one foot as you sway, and set it back down several inches to the front, back, or side, so your weight transfers completely to one foot and then the other.

Being rigid only creates an illusion of balance. True balance is the ability to move in any direction, at any moment.

Ferris Wheel

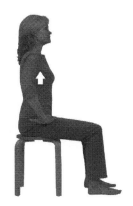 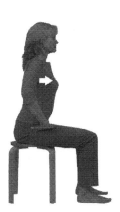 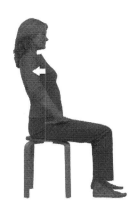

A droopy chest is the hallmark of poor posture. In a belly dance class, my stunning teacher, Aleili, taught an exercise that I've adapted to mobilize the rib cage and strengthen the muscles between the shoulder blades. Practice this and turn droopy into perky.

1   Sit in a chair with your feet and your sit bones planted firmly and evenly. Put your hands on your hips.

2   Lift your ribcage up, as far away from your pelvis as possible. Return to neutral. Repeat five times.

3   Push your chest forward as far as possible, and then draw it back to slightly behind neutral. Repeat this motion five times.

4   To create your Ferris wheel, slide your ribcage forward, up, over the top; then release it down in the back and then forward again. Think of a Ferris wheel picking up passengers at the bottom and carrying them up and around. Make up to 10 revolutions.

5   Change directions. At the top of your revolution, send your ribcage forward, then down, back, and up over the top for an equal number of circles.

6   Alternate between forward and backward revolutions. Vary the point at which you change directions.

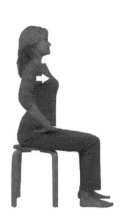 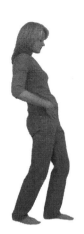 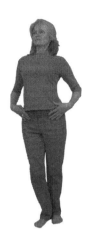

7 Relax, and allow your hips, legs, and arms to follow the movement. Stand if you prefer.

8 Sit or lie down to rest. If your body wants to twitch or wiggle, let it. You don't need be still to rest; just be at peace.

Variation #1

ॐ Stand and perform the undulation. To stabilize your pelvis so it doesn't wobble, let your knees be flexible, place one foot slightly ahead of the other, and draw your belly button to your spine.

Variation #2

ॐ Add a lean to the left and right. Place your left foot six to eight inches ahead of the right. Point your ribcage over the forward toe and undulate. Reverse your feet and the angle of your ribcage; undulate to the right.

*Discovering new **internal** places may enliven your **external** outlook.*

Chicken Walk

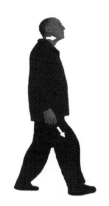 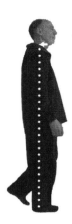 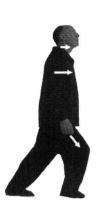 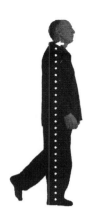

This undulation actually emphasizes a bad habit that many of us share—the head forward posture. By consciously connecting this to walking, you can loosen your neck and bring it back over your body. It also strengthens an important component of your stride, when one leg supports your entire weight.

1 Find a place where you can walk uninterrupted. It's OK to walk around the living room, but change directions so it's not always the same circle.

2 Walk slowly.

3 As one leg swings forward, reach forward with your chin and neck up to one inch.

4 As you put weight on that leg, pull your chin and neck back so your head is directly over your body and in line with your torso, pelvis and leg.

5 Continue in this manner; jut your face forward and back, in coordination with your stride. Your head will bob forward and back, like a chicken.

6 Add your chest and connect the movements of your torso and neck, so they both move forward and back over your legs.

7 Don't overdo this one; five minutes is plenty of time to get the benefit. Going too long can strain weak neck muscles.

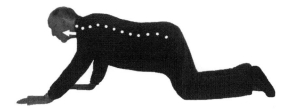 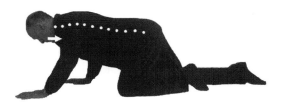

8 Finish with a normal walk. Feel for the natural undulations. (See the Walking undulation on pages 58 and 59.)

9 Stand or sit to rest. Notice how your head is aligned over your neck, pelvis, and feet.

Variation #1

This variation is called "The Turtle."

- Crawl around, preferably on a soft surface like a carpeted floor.

- Like a turtle peeking out of its shell, jut your chin forward about a half an inch, as you reach with each arm.

- As you bring weight onto each arm, pull your neck back so that it is in line with the rest of your spine. Feel the stretch along the back of your neck.

- Continue bobbing your neck as you crawl for a few minutes.

*There is a fine line between the pain of injury and
that of working outside your normal pattern.
Be mindful of what is out of bounds for you.*

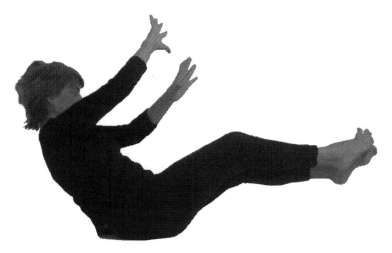

For the Core

When you think of a strong core, do you visualize six-pack abs and muscled bodies in skimpy clothes? Core muscles don't show on the outside. They are the deep muscles closest to the skeleton, designed to stabilize your bones. Think of an apple core; you can't see that through the skin.

Not only are core muscles deep, but many of them are small so they respond best to small and slow movements. These undulations might not look like your typical core exercises, but trust me, you'll feel these inner muscles develop. Skimpy clothes not required.

Blooming Lotus

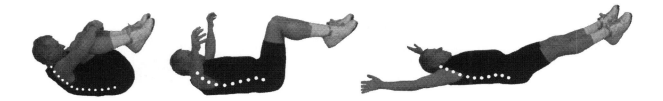

Exercise is half sit-up and half just goofing around. I find myself regularly popping it into my morning Free Form practice. My body likes it—as though I am blooming, one petal at a time, into the day.

1   Lie on your back. Bring your knees up above your hips and lift your feet off the floor.

2   Lift your head and chest slowly toward your knees. Wrap your arms around your legs and make yourself into a ball.

3   Once you reach your maximum curl, open up and stretch out all your limbs.

4   When your head touches the floor, curl up into a ball again.

5   Use one limb at a time to reach out and back. Return to your curl between each. Spread out again.

6   Move your arms and legs randomly in and out.

7   Curl up only part way.

8   Expand and contract differently each time.

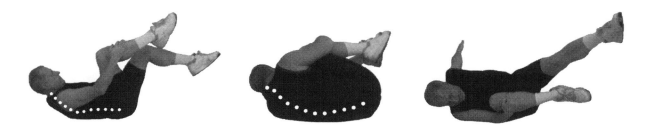

9   Add angles and rolls and merge into Free Form.

10   Rest in any comfortable position until your breath returns to its normal rhythm.

Variation #1

    ❧ Do this undulation series on your side.

You can easily connect to other people and the world around you when you are in touch with your internal self.

Coffee Grinder

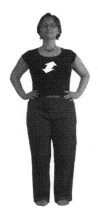 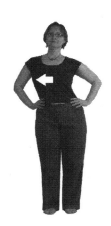 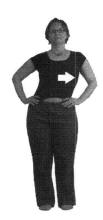

This undulation creates strong abdominal muscles and the idea you might be able to grind coffee beans with your midsection. It's no coincidence that my chiropractor and fellow belly dance sister has this spine-twisting move down pat.

1. Stand with your hands on your hips.

2. Push your ribcage forward as far as possible; then slide it back to slightly behind neutral. Hold your hips still. Repeat this five times.

3. Slide your ribcage to the right and then through center to the left. Glide side-to-side with stable hips five times.

4. Combine the movements to make a diamond pattern. Move your ribcage forward, right, back, left, and then forward again. Draw your diamond parallel to the floor.

5. Repeat the motion, but round the corners to draw a circle parallel to the floor.

6. After a few times clockwise, go counter-clockwise.

7. Add your hips. As your ribs slide right, shift your hips left and vice versa. Go back and forth several times.

8. Combine the chest circles and hip circles:

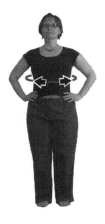 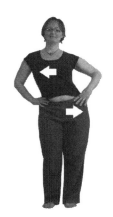 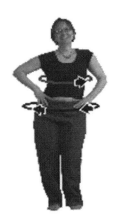

- Slide your ribs to the right and hips to the left;
- Push your ribs forward and bring your hips back to neutral;
- Slide your ribs to the left and hips to the right;
- Return all parts to neutral.

9 Continue for a minute with your ribs going clockwise and the hips providing a counterbalance.

10 Reverse directions for a minute.

11 Let go of your torso-hip connection and allow your body to work out its own kinks in Free Form.

12 Sit to rest. Feel the strength of your midsection. Notice the entire front of your spine.

Variation #1

- Make small circles with your neck–opposite of your chest. Go both ways.
- Gyrate all over and allow your neck, ribs, and pelvis to circle independently of each other.
- Keep everything small and controlled.

Be aware of where you are.
Start from there—with the simple intention to improve.

Swing

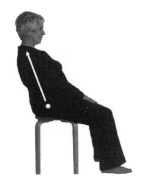 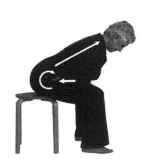 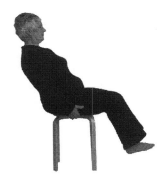

Do you remember the childish joy of swinging? Ah, the wind in your hair, the air under your legs and that wonderful feeling of flight. Now I feel foolish if I even sit on a playground swing. What a shame we think swinging is only for children! This easy, fun and active undulation keeps the body walking longer.

1 Sit on the edge of a sturdy chair. Keep your back straight and feet on the floor.

2 Lean your torso back and then forward. Move from your hips joints and keep your spine long. (Don't let it bend.)

3 Put your fingers in the crease at the front of your hip joints. Lean your upper body forward and fold over your fingers like the flap of a cardboard box. Open up and away as you lean back and unfold.

4 Hold onto the sides of the chair by your thighs so you can add your legs.

5 Lift your feet from the floor and straighten your legs slightly as you lean back.

6 Bend your knees as you return upright and lean forward.

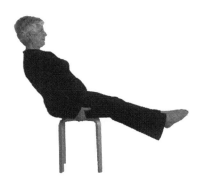 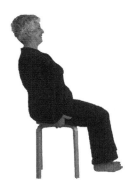 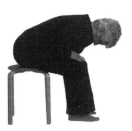

7 Coordinate the movement of your legs and body like you are on a swing. Let the movement flow from your legs and up through your spine.

8 After swinging for several minutes, add other movements such as rotation and side bending to turn this into a Free Form undulation.

9 Sit for a minute and rest. Smile.

Variation #1

❧ Find a park with swings–ignore that self-consciousness–and swing. Lean back and look at the sky or react passively to the rocking motion. Either way, your joints will benefit.

Variation #2

❧ Sit on a chair and lean forward so that your chest touches your thighs.

❧ Press through your feet and use your buttocks to push your chest up. Roll yourself upright and back to a sitting position.

❧ Arch your back slightly and fold forward until your chest touches your legs again.

❧ Repeat the above steps.

How did you play as a child?
Give yourself permission to try some of your former favorite activities.

Eel

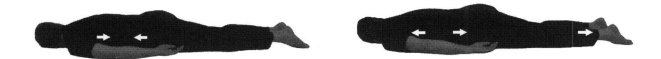

This undulation will teach you to use the intricacies of your spine by slithering. Eels have powerful, strong cores, because that's all they have. Eels can't fall back on arms and legs.

1. Lie facedown on the floor, arms at your sides, legs and feet together. You can turn your head to one side or have your forehead on the floor; which ever is comfortable for your neck.

2. Pull your left shoulder and hip toward each other. Then push them as far apart as possible. Reach down with your foot and hip to improve the length of your stretch.

3. As you expand on the left side, enhance the contraction on your right by scrunching your right shoulder and hip toward each other.

4. Now push your right hip and shoulder apart and reach with your right foot.

5. Alternate sides. As you move between shortening and lengthening, notice the wave that travels up or down your spine.

6. Let the image of an eel's easy, slinky locomotion guide your movement, whether you move along the ground or not.

7. Release yourself from the confines of being *an eel*. Take the new knowledge of your core and let it lead your Free Form undulation.

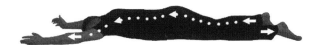

8 Rest; stand with a newfound appreciation for being upright.

Variation #1

- ❧ Start in the same face-down position on the floor. Reach overhead and try to touch your fingers together. Also, keep your legs and feet together.

- ❧ Stretch the arm and foot on one side apart as the other side contracts.

- ❧ Reverse and repeat.

Variation #2

- ❧ Undulate at angles to the right or left rather than straight ahead.

- ❧ Try variations in the reach and coordination between your spine and limbs.

- ❧ Have fun with it!

Remember that small movements can be powerful;
they often activate neglected muscles.

Caressed by Waves

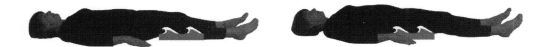

In this exercise, you'll engage the intrinsic muscles of your back by *floating* on the lift of a wave. Think of this as a Zen, doing-less-is-more exercise, since the movements are small and slow.

1 Lie on your back. If your low back complains, put a long flat pillow lengthwise under each leg, so your legs are inclined and knees straight.

2 Imagine lying on warm, sandy beach at the water's edge, your feet pointing at the ocean. The rolling surf lifts you in a gentle wave, from your feet, to your legs, then hips, and up under your spine.

3 Recreate this gentle undulation with your muscles. Roll the wave up and then back down your spine. Include your arms.

4 Your imagination controls this exercise, unless you have a recording of waves to guide you. Incorporate different wave intervals and intensities.

5 Change the direction of the waves. Flow from one foot, up to the opposite shoulder, and back. Continue for several minutes.

6 Change course into a Free Form undulation that expresses your body's current desire for movement.

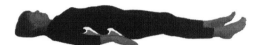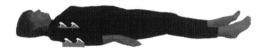

7 Lie still. Breathe; be conscious of the natural waves inside you.

Variation #1

    ⁜ Imagine floating in the middle of the sea. Use your muscles to create the sensations of riding the swells and gentle bobbing.

Tune into your body's natural harmony:
pulse–brain waves–breath–lymph flow–digestion–craniosacral rhythm.

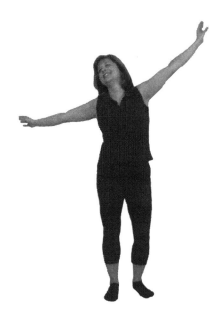

Chapter Three

Characteristics of a

Youthful Body

YOU KNOW THE OLD CHILDREN'S VERSE about how the body is connected? The foot bone's connected to the leg bone; the leg bone's connected to the thigh bone . . . the neck bone's connected to the head bone. This implies that our bones are stacked on top of one other like the bricks of a building. But if your bones were actually rubbing together—ouch—like bricks missing mortar between them, the joints would have degenerated causing you a lot of grinding pain.

Misunderstanding how our bodies work is a major reason we don't use them optimally. And misinformation is more detrimental than lack of motivation or time constraints, in my opinion. So in this chapter, I'll give you basic information on the relevant parts of the body that you'll be using in these exercises.

I'll explain the fundamentals of body structure; giving you better idea of what to look for or what you may feel as you go through the undulations, which types of movement add fluidity, and which could increase stiffness. You'll learn what creates health, causes injury, and how to care for yourself. Also, you'll gain a better understanding of how your body is built, how many ways it can move, and just how alive it can feel.

Joints and Connective Tissue

Your bones connect through your joints. They are held together—and apart—by connective tissue. This term includes ligaments, tendons, muscles, cartilage, and fascia, the very matrix that determines your body's shape. Connective tissue facilitates or inhibits every movement you make. For joints to function optimally, the matrix must be balanced and fluid, equally strong and flexible. When part of the connective tissue matrix is tighter than others, force is distributed unequally through the joints increasing the risk of injury.

Cartilage

Did you know that the primary component of cartilage is water? It's true—60 to 75 percent! Another interesting fact about cartilage is that it's a major component of the discs between your vertebrae. Cartilage has no direct blood flow, so it depends on the movement of fluid produced by physical activity for nutrients and removal of waste products. Regular exercise is particularly important, because cartilage thins with age and lack of use. It can be damaged by connective tissue irregularities or compression, increasing the risk of osteoarthritis.

Bones

Even the hardest parts of our bodies, the bones, are more fluid than most of us imagine. Healthy, living bone is porous and has elastic qualities. Cells continually lay down new bone structure and remodel new tissue. You may think of bones as petrified, but they're really a dynamic and ever-changing part of our bodies.

The Spine

There are 24 separate vertebrae in your neck and back, plus the sacrum and tailbone. (Figure 3.1 shows a spine and individual vertebra. Figure 3.2 shows a vertebra, top view.) Your spine includes the entire length, from head to tail. Each individual segment has the ability to rotate, move forward and backward, *and* side-to-side. That's 24 different places you can move your spine—in a lot of various ways.

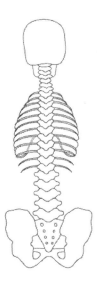

Figure 3.1. Back view of spine including the skull, ribs, and pelvis.
Note there are 24 vertebrae plus the sacrum and tailbone,
providing a myriad number of places to move.

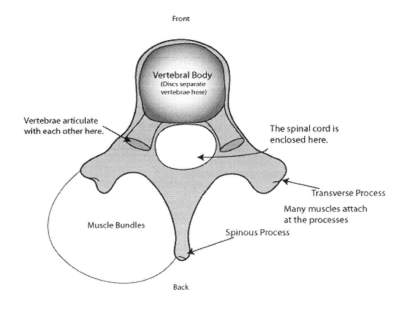

Figure 3.2. Each vertebra (top view shown) provides multiple places for articulation,
muscle attachment and protection for the spinal cord.

When you bend over, those bumps that poke up are the back of your vertebrae. While we may consider these the "back bone," each one is actually up to several inches deep. The front of each vertebra is nearer to the center of your body than you might think. As a matter of fact, did you know that the common, protruding hump at the base of the neck in the back could be caused by tight connective tissue in the front?

Muscles

Muscles are arranged throughout the body in layers. Core muscles—those closest to bone—stabilize your skeleton. They provide the foundation for balance, help prevent injury, and produce slow, fine motions. Core muscles often get frozen or stuck from lack of use. When this happens, other muscles must work two jobs, stabilizing the body and moving themselves at the same time. It's a conflict of interest that causes muscular tension and makes them especially susceptible to strain.

> The core muscles around your spine are small muscles—many less than an inch long—and connect the vertebra to one another. There are many different angles of attachments, which creates a profound capacity for movement.

In addition, the outer layers of muscle reach all the way up your spine with tendrils that attach to each rib and vertebra. If the tendrils retain uneven tension, portions of the back can become too short and others too long. (See Figure 3.3 and 3.4 for examples.) Undulation can help you discover and correct muscle and tissue imbalances.

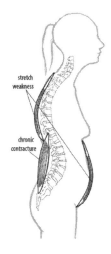

Figure 3.3.
A scoliosis is supported by short muscles.
(Reprinted with kind permissiony of Mary Ann Foster from
Somatic Patterning, EMS Press 2004)

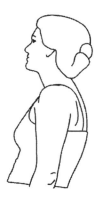

Figure 3.4.
Chronically short and long muscles create poor posture.

Take a moment to feel your back while you sway. How many different joints can you feel moving? If you're like most of us, movement is probably confined to only a few vertebrae. Our goal, of course, is to be able to move each independently, in all three planes of movement (rotate, forward and back, side to side). When more of the spine is involved, the coordinated small movement of each vertebra adds up to one large, easy motion.

Taking Care of Your Muscles

I encourage you to drink plenty of water, which is required for good health. Even though your muscles need fluid to stay supple, your internal organs get higher priority. When you're not fully hydrated, fluid will seep from your muscles and connective tissue, drying up their supply of nutrients and making removal of waste difficult.

While getting enough fluid into your body might be the first step, getting it into the muscles is the second.

> Muscular activity regulates much of the flow
> of liquid throughout your system.

When it contracts, a muscle forces fluid from the surrounding connective tissue. As it relaxes, fresh, available fluid flows back in. A muscle can become dehydrated and dry out like beef jerky if it's chronically contracted. It may also start grabbing nearby tissue for some temporary additional strength, causing adhesions that can later constrict movement.

Without fresh fluid from regular use, a muscle can become stagnant. A brace-like structure may develop when the connective tissue lays down extra fibers to support the immobility. Asking a muscle to contract with all that extra fortification is like asking a piece of plywood to bend. A "tight" muscle may actually need to be shortened instead of stretched like you may think. For example, in the habitual rolled-forward posture (shown in Figure 3.4) the upper back, neck, and shoulders are elongated, but stretching these tissues actually creates more stiffness, not less.

Undulation works to get fluid back into and soften dehydrated tissues, adhesions and wooden muscles.

Snap, Crackle and Pop

Do you make noise when you move? Inactivity can cause tight tendons or hard crystals in the tissues that sound downright cranky! Maybe you're worried that these noises are bones rubbing together, but that wouldn't be just cranky; it would be excruciating. Moving—without pain—is the best thing you can do for these tissues. It helps to lengthen tendons and reabsorb those crunchy crystals.

Injuries

Even though undulation is intended to help you heal, it's still possible to injure yourself with any new activity. Avoid soft-tissue damage; don't push too hard or fast. Injuries are rare though, if you stay fully conscious of where your body is and what you're doing with it. Have faith that you'll make progress with consistent, gentle work.

I divide injuries into two major categories: overstretch and overuse.

Overstretch Injuries

If you stretch too far, you can actually create tears within muscle and connective tissue. These tiny lacerations get repaired with scar tissue, which by nature's design, is inflexible and stiff. Going for the "burn" is too much and counterproductive. ***Stretching is most effective done only to the point of first sensation, which requires an awareness of subtle changes.***

Overstretch injuries can also happen when we aren't even aware of them. Sitting slumped on the couch or during a long car ride can overstretch ligaments in the low back. Breaking up a static position with little movements like undulations can help. Ergonomic experts recommend moving every 20 minutes.

Overuse Injuries

Unless you were a prodigy, you probably didn't learn math all at once. But for some reason, we all want our bodies to do the physical equivalent of calculus right out of the starting gate. It just isn't possible. And when we try, try again, an injury from overuse is usually the result. A much more effective long-term strategy is to build up your strength gradually and let muscles rest after intense activity.

Another common cause of injury is using one part of the body more than it is designed for, such as bending at one vertebra, rather than spreading the movement over several, or over-rotating the neck, because the torso does not. The tissues around these overworked areas soon become worn out and exhausted. By learning to use your whole body, these types of injuries are preventable.

In Conclusion

Did you know that your body tries to duplicate mental imagery? If you imagine your body as a mechanical framework with a rigid structure, it will inevitably, literally think itself stiff. A healthier vision might be to consider your many moving parts as living components of one organism. Nourish it with movement and attention.

Remember, you're not only what you eat, but what you do as well.

Your body and all of its parts conform to how you use them. If you feel your body is limiting your current activities, it may be time to—gently—build in new range of motion. I can't think of any better exercise than undulation, because it builds strength and flexibility deep within the spine.

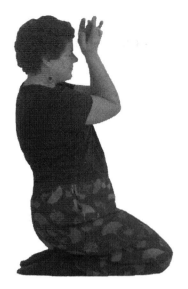

For Scoliosis

Scoliosis ranges from mild to severe and can be caused by a short leg, uneven pelvis, or no known cause (idiopathic). Most people with scoliosis are highly functional and the spine curvature is more of an annoyance, if noticed at all, than any type of disability. There are no known cures for scoliosis, but several methods do reduce spinal curvature. Even without a formal scoliosis, many people have asymmetry in the sides of their torso. The following exercises are designed to help you achieve more even range of motion and strength on both sides of your spine, important components of improving function and reducing susceptibility to injury.

Bellows

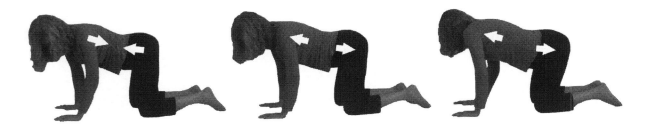

Like a bellows that fuels a fire with air, your side can pump energy into your discs and muscles, vitalize your breath, and tighten your waist.

1 Get on your hands and knees.

2 Warm up with a minute of Free Form undulation.

3 Inhale. Draw your left shoulder and hip together in a contraction. Use the pressure to build internal energy.

4 Exhale. Stretch your left shoulder and hip as far apart as possible. Force all the pent up energy out.

5 Repeat the inhale/contraction and exhale/stretch on your right side.

6 Alternate sides, repeat five times on both.

7 Now try the opposite; exhale as you contract and inhale as you stretch. Which breathing pattern helps you to create energy and which helps you to relax?

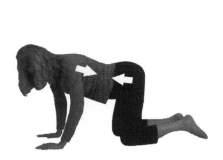
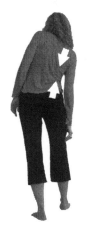
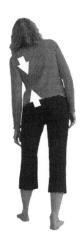

8   Coordinate the movements; as one side lengthens, contract the other at the same time. Then reverse.

9   Add other movements to your side-bend; progress into Free Form.

10   Sit or lie down. Rest until your breath has steadied and your energy is calm.

Variation #1

❦ Do this undulation lying on your back.

Variation #2

❦ Walk; and side bend over the leg bearing your weight.

Movement is your internal water and energy pump.

Barber Pole

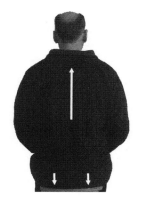 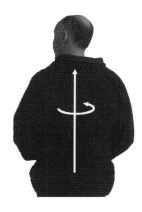 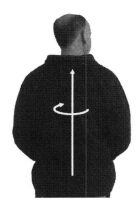

This undulation is an excellent exercise for your core—which must engage to support your straight spine—and for your back muscles—which are responsible for coordinating the twist. Core strength is necessary to be able to rotate without compensating by side bending or shifting.

1   Sit on a chair with both feet firmly on the floor. This can also be done sitting on the floor if your hips are flexible, but try a chair first.

2   As you inhale, press your feet down in to the floor and your sit bones down into the chair. Slightly lift your spine and ribs.

3   Exhale—stay tall and twist your spine to the right. Imagine your spine as a barber pole, revolving around the center.

4   Try not to let your sit bones lift, your side collapse, or your ribs shift to either side as you twist.

5   Inhale and unwind the twist. Exhale as you return to the twist.

6   Notice if one part twists more than another (neck, shoulders, etc.). If so, limit the movement in that area to match the rest of your spine.

7   Repeat the sequence, twisting to the left.

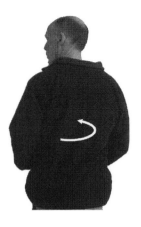 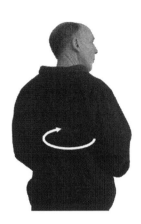 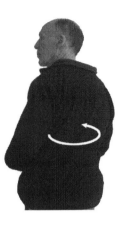

8 After twisting both ways several times each, let your spine move in a different direction, especially forward and back.

9 Rest for a minute until your spine comes to a place of tranquility.

Variation #1

- ❧ Twist and untwist so that it takes five counts to get to the back of the twist and another five counts to return. Do this a few times to each side. Then use a count of 10 for both sides a few times.

- ❧ Now slow it down even more. Say the alphabet as you twist, starting from neutral at "A" and ending at the back of the twist at "Z." Return at this same, slow pace. Hint: aim for "M" at your halfway point.

Variation #2

- ❧ As you twist, let you arms hang naturally with your hands relaxed at your sides or resting in your lap. Wind and unwind, keeping your arms totally relaxed (pretend they are asleep) so that all the motion is coming from the

Remember the goal is not necessarily to twist to the fullest.
The intention is to become more aware of your body.

Mermaid

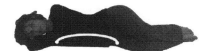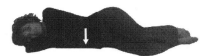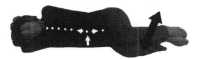

The Mermaid came from trying to simulate swimming on my bedroom floor after I realized that we might be more fluid if we swam more. Note that your body will move differently when you're on your side.

1   Lie on the floor on your side with both legs bent. Support your head with your hand, arm or pillow.

2   Notice that your hip and shoulder press against the floor more firmly than your waist does.

3   At the waist, press your spine toward the floor and distribute the weight evenly between your waist and ribs.

4   Let your waist return to its normal curve and allow the ripple to extend throughout your body. Repeat a few times.

5   Now try it from your hip. Press your waist to the floor by rolling your top hip in and up toward the ceiling.

6   Come back to neutral.

7   Sw*im* your legs from the hip down–together, like a mermaid swimming– and allow the movement to follow through your torso and shoulders. Swim for a minute.

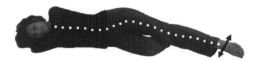 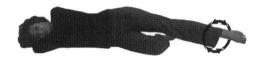

8   Turn onto your other side and repeat the entire sequence.

9   Roll on your back and bring your knees toward your chest. Undulate as a ball for a minute.

10   Straighten your legs (put a pillow under your knees if needed for your low back) and rest. Let all sensations sink from your body into the ground.

Variation #1

- ❧ Lie on your side with your bottom leg bent and top leg straight.

- ❧ Move the straight leg forward and back a few inches. Let the waves follow through your entire spine and out your head.

- ❧ Now move that leg in small circles, clockwise and counterclockwise so your spine and head oscillate. Repeat for a minute or so.

- ❧ Try both ways at different speeds.

- ❧ Roll on your other side and repeat.

Include daily variety and add new moves regularly
to keep your body supple.

Sideways Roll

 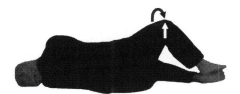

The goal of this exercise is to build vigor in your hips and core muscles. Resist the urge to go for the burn when stretching. Instead, focus on the balance between your flexibility and strength.

1   Lie on your side with your knees and hips bent. Use pillows for your neck if needed, one on each side. (Isn't this a great exercise already? You get to lie in a typical sleeping position!)

2   Take a moment to truly rest.

3   Slowly increase the space between your knees by bringing your top knee up in an arc, leaving your feet together. At some point, the pull on your pelvis will draw your body and leg over to the other side.

4   Rest again briefly.

5   Repeat the knee lift and roll from this side.

6   Check in often with your back for any soreness. If you find any, rest for a minute before continuing. If you still feel sore, that's enough for one day.

7   Move slowly so you can feel the muscles around your hip rotate your thigh. Use the muscles in your back to support your body. Keep the movement soft and flowing. Do about 10 rolls.

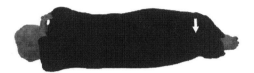 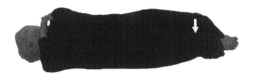

8   Add an undulation on each side for several seconds and let your momentum carry you through the roll.

9   Lie comfortably on your back with knees bent or straight. Let the newly created energy in your pelvis drain away.

Variation #1

- Lie on your back with your knees bent, feet on the floor, and arms out to the sides. (Place large pillows or couch cushions right next to your legs if your hips are tight.)

- Let your right knee fall out to the right side. Follow with your left leg; bring your left knee down to rest on your right calf. Keep your shoulders as flat as possible on the floor throughout the movement.

- Keep your shoulders on the floor and reverse the motion; arc your left knee up and over first, and follow it with the right.

- Roll from side to side. Initiate the leg movements from your hips and follow along with your low back while your upper back stays flat.

Draw your belly button in toward your spine to engage your core abdominal muscles. This will stabilize and protect your back.

Figure 8

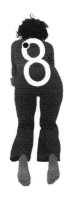 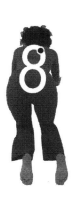 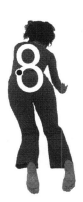

Here's an opportunity to coordinate your upper and lower body. This exercise is challenging or fun–depending on the attitude you bring to it. Either way, prepare to be amused.

1 Get on your hands and knees.

2 Move your chest to the left and *up* toward your chin. Circle your chest around to the right and back *down* to where you started.

3 As you reach your starting position, move your low back and hips to the left and *down* toward your tailbone. Then circle it around to the right and back *up* to the starting position again.

4 You have just made a figure 8 with your torso.

5 Continue the circulation of movement between your upper and lower torso. Make the size of your size of your 8's bigger and smaller.

6 Reverse so that your upper torso curves to the right. Continue until you feel balanced.

7 Lead with your hips in both directions.

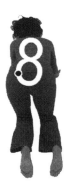 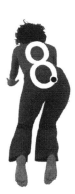

8 Lose the definition of the figure 8 as your body follows its own lead in Free Form.

9 In a seated position, let go of all tension and enjoy the flexibility you have just created.

Variation #1

❧ Bring your torso closer to and away from the floor as you circle around so that you create different angles of movement.

Variation #2

❧ Do this undulation very, very slowly to strengthen your core. Work toward having each cycle last a full minute.

How many shapes can you make
with how many different parts of your body?

_____
_____
_____
_____
_____
_____
_____
_____
_____
_____
_____
_____
_____
_____
_____
_____
_____
_____
_____
_____
_____
_____
_____
_____
_____
_____
_____
_____

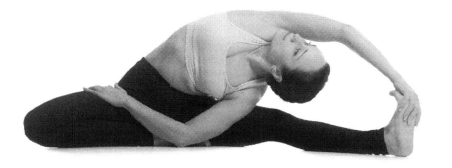

For Hypermobility

Being very flexible seems like a novelty to children, but over time it can lead to instability in the joints and create a host of problems later in life. A strong core is essential to protect the joints, especially the many joints of the spine. People with hypermobility have a talent for large movements—big stretches and fast recoil. Being able to concentrate and sustain tiny, slow movements and to connect different parts of the body can seem tedious or even impossible at first, but with a little practice these undulations will help pull the skeleton together.

Tree Tops

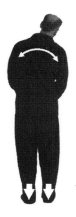 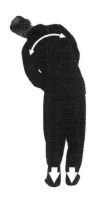 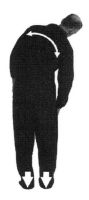

Like people, trees are living organisms, not mechanical devices. Even the strongest trees must undulate; they'd break if they didn't. Notice the trees in your environment and duplicate their motions.

1   Stand with your feet directly under your hips. If you have balance difficulties, stand by a wall or have a sturdy chair handy for support. Look at, or just imagine, trees.

2   Get grounded. Feel the bottoms of your feet and what's underneath them. Is it concrete or wooden framing? How far under your feet is the earth? What is the soil like 10 feet down?

3   Now that you've *grown* your roots, remove all bracing from your upper body so that it can lean and sway. When you feel off balance, focus on the connection between your feet and the ground and bring yourself back to center.

4   Imagine a gentle wind blowing through your branches. Move with your imaginary breeze as it shifts directions.

5   Imagine you are many different types of trees: oak, redwood, palm. Notice how your equilibrium adjusts to the various shapes and features.

6   Stay grounded as you widen your stance to achieve a more pronounced undulation. Encourage your body to choose the Free Form most beneficial for you today.

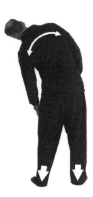 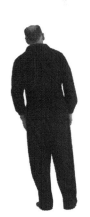 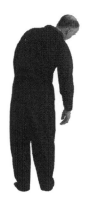

7   Transition your feet gradually from being planted to being mobile.

8   Walk slowly as a form of rest. Give your feet the opportunity to undulate before you return to your other daily activities.

Variation #1

    ೭ Imagine your feet are rooted in soft mud. Let your legs, hips, torso and arms float–like seaweed in the ocean currents.

As you become more accomplished at undulation,
you'll find that balance is not rigid; it's fluid.

Unnoticeable

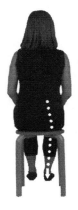 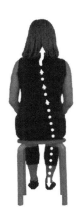 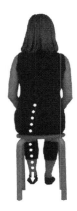

Tiny, unnoticeable movements engage the intrinsic muscles of your spine: often neglected and literally less than an inch long. This technique can keep your spine engaged and fluid all day long even if you're on an airplane or stuck in a long meeting.

1   Sit with your feet and sit bones well grounded.

2   Press the heel and ball of one foot into the ground. Feel the force travel up your leg, hips, and low back.

3   Carry the minuscule wave on up your spine and through your neck.

4   Release the pressure from your foot and control the gradual movement back to neutral.

5   Repeat the press, wave, and release with your other foot.

6   Alternate side-to-side, like a cat kneading its paws. Use 10 second or more for each side. Focus on the continuity through all parts of your back and try to keep the shift at your shoulders to less than half an inch

7   Now, with your sit bones anchored and feet engaged, but not pushing, keep the tiny movements rolling.

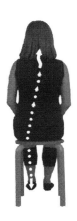 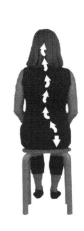 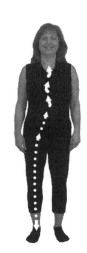

8 Keep everything very small and slow.

9 As you rest, notice that stillness is not stationary. Your heart still moves blood. Your lungs still move oxygen. Being alive equals movement!

Variation #1

& Try this while you stand in line at the grocery store or as you wait for the gas tank to fill.

When your whole body contributes to movement,
no single part is over-stressed.

Back Massage

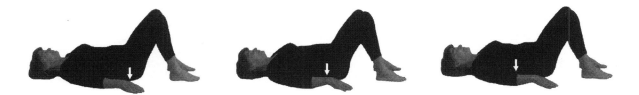

Everyone loves a good back rub. Here you'll learn to use your core muscles in conjunction with gravity to bring relief to those stiff spots, increase your circulation and unwind. No appointment needed—and it's free!

1   Lie on your back on a hard surface with knees bent and feet on the ground.

2   Press your tailbone to the floor for a count of three and release.

3   Press your sacrum to the floor for a count of three and release.

4   Press your right hip to the floor; count three and release. Then three counts with your left hip, release.

5   Progress up your back about two inches at a time; press one side down and then the other. Hold each for a count of three and rest in between.

6   When you get to the top of your shoulder blades, go back to get any spots that feel missed. Hold the pressure for the amount of time that feels right for that place.

7   Wriggle around in different directions: lift off the floor, press into it, twist, turn, and roll. Enjoy that your body can move as well as it does.

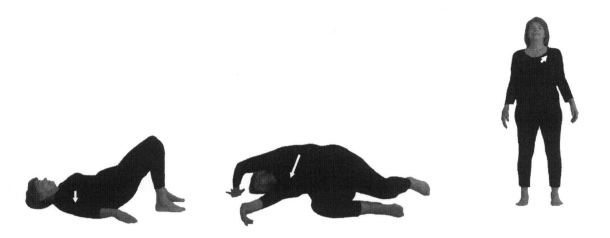

8 Lie on your tummy for a short time to rest. Imagine any remaining tension floating away into the air.

Variation #1

Now move a bit faster so that you roll up and down and across your back, rather than holding and releasing. Do what feels good.

Variation #2

 ✎ Repeat the hold and release sequence standing against a wall.

Every body is built differently, so not every exercise will come easily.
Be kind to yourself if it's difficult.

Train Cars

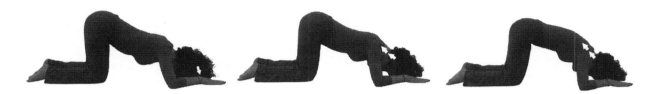

The objective of this undulation is to transfer movement from one vertebra to the next. Think of your vertebrae like boxcars in a train: each one separate, but also connected. When the engine pulls or pushes the first car, it then pulls or pushes the second car and so on, all the way to the caboose. This undulation was inspired by an exercise in *Making Connections* by Peggy Hackney.

1   On your hands and knees, rest your forearms and forehead on the floor.

2   Push your forehead into the ground with curiosity. Find the spot between the crown of your head and eyebrows that best transfers the movement along your neck.

3   Gently press this spot and feel each vertebra in your neck articulate sequentially.

4   Try again if you don't feel the articulation at first.

5   After you begin to feel the vertebrae in your neck push each other, continue the locomotion down your back—from vertebra to vertebra.

6   The sensation of this movement is subtle. It could feel like the spread of warmth, opening of space, or the flow of water down your spine. Accentuate whatever you sense with vivid mental imagery.

7   When you feel the movement stop or skip, rest and begin again from the top. Each time, you may incorporate another and another vertebra. Movement will inch from the back of your skull, through your neck, down your back, and out through your tail.

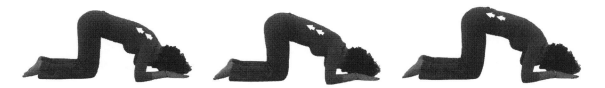

8 It may take many times for the motion to travel down your entire spine, and still, some places may get derailed. Be patient and gentle.

9 Repeat the full length of your spine—or as far as you can go—up to 10 times.

10 Morph into a Free Form undulation.

11 Lie on your back and feel the continuous movements of your breath and spine.

Variation #1

• Get on your hands and knees. Keep your head level with your shoulders.

• Tuck your tail under so your low back arches up toward the ceiling and your lumbar vertebrae flex. From this position, your sacrum will push on the lowest lumbar vertebra which will then push the one above it.

• After you can feel your low back move vertebra to vertebra, continue the movement up your back to your skull.

Imagining a sensation is often the first step in feeling it.

Whirlpool

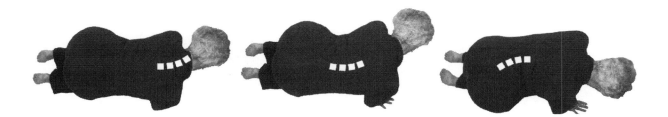

This exercise creates a whirlpool that swirls around as easily as water down the bathtub drain. As in the *Train Cars* undulation, the object is to transfer movement directly from one vertebra to the next, but now with soft angles merged in.

1. Get on your hands and knees, hands directly under your shoulders and knees directly under your hips.

2. Tilt your head to the left a couple inches and follow with your neck. Imagine the right sides of the spaces between each vertebra spreading open.

3. When the bend reaches the base of your neck, stop the head movement and focus on your back. Let each vertebra nudge the next and the next, like dominoes in slow motion, and allow your weight to shift right.

4. Bring your weight back to center gradually, using each segment of your low back in turn.

5. Point your tailbone to the right and keep moving. Allow the low back vertebrae to open, one by one, to the left.

6. Shift your weight to the left and let your head tilt to the right.

7. From your mid-back (not your neck), move each upper back and neck segment closer to center in sequence and bring your head back to neutral.

Undulation: Relieve Stiffness and Feel Young

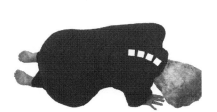 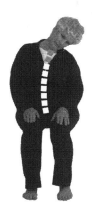 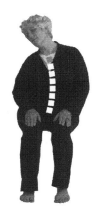

8 Continue clockwise for several revolutions; then change directions for equal balance.

9 Introduce arches and folds into the whirlpool to create Free Form movements. Stand up for variety.

10 Rest seated, reflecting on the concept of your back as an integrated and cooperative whole.

Variation #1

❧ Reverse the swirl from the top, bottom or sides. The interruption of momentum will help you develop those hard-to-reach, intrinsic muscles. Don't avoid the weak spots—zero in on them.

Variation #2

❧ Sit and try this undulation. Gravity will be a weightier factor.

You can easily connect to other people and the world around you when you are in touch with your internal self.

Notes

Undulation: Relieve Stiffness and Feel Young

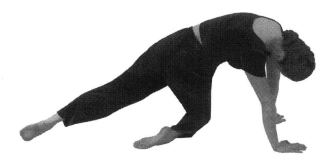

To Enhance Body Awareness

Body awareness isn't valued much and is often seen as something superfluous to everyday tasks. On the contrary, body awareness plays a vital role in our ability to accurately interpret our sensations, draw conclusions from the environment around us, even to balance. That being said, these undulations require a bit of imagination and willingness to feel inside. If you already have a practice where you tune in regularly to your sensations, you can jump right in. If not, don't get discouraged if you are frustrated at first. It took me years to develop the awareness to be able to feel things so subtle.

Speed Bump

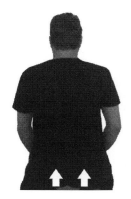 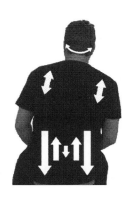 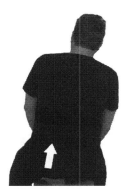

This exercise teaches you how to let go of unconscious tension held in your body. Habitual stiffness prevents natural movement when driving on a bumpy road or when staying still on a turbulent airplane flight; and this reinforces the tension. Learn to stay fluid and float through those bumps of life.

1   Sit in a chair and imagine driving over a speed bump.

2   Use your legs to lift your buttocks off the seat a half an inch. Plop back down.

3   Let the bounce echo through your body. Notice how many times your shoulders wiggle and head wobbles. Allow a full five seconds for the effects to dissipate.

4   Lift again—but push on your left leg a little harder than the right. When you release, you'll come down at a slight angle and the effect will travel differently through your torso.

5   Now push a little harder with your right foot. Alternate sides and repeat 10 times.

6   Change how you start the bump often and allow enough time for your muscles to soften.

7   Exaggerate the plop if your neck can handle abrupt movement.

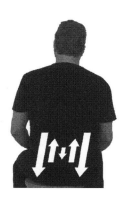 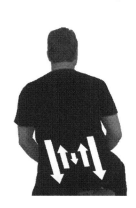 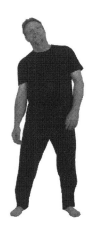

8   Take your ride out of the parking lot and onto a bumpy road. Bounce and
     sway in the seat to imitate the jostle of gravel and the jolt of small
     potholes.

9   Drive into a Free Form undulation. Smooth out any rough edges this
     exercise may have produced.

10   Rest. Be aware of your center and take a moment to enjoy the idea of not
     going anywhere for a minute.

Variation #1

   ❧ Stand as though you are on a boat. Use your legs and upper body to adjust to
     and compensate for the churning, choppy water.

Variation #2

   ❧ Sit. With your hips, simulate the effects of being on flight battered by
     turbulence and let the rest of your body follow.

Build strength and flexibility equally
for well-balanced health.

Sprocket Wheel

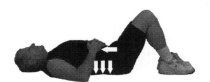 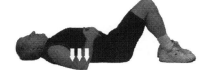 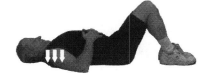

You'll use the floor to improve your spine's mobility and develop its intrinsic muscles during this undulation. Use caution if you have a history or a suspicion of disc problems. The way to assure long-lasting results is to build strength and flexibility slowly.

1   Lie on your back with legs bent and feet on the floor.

2   The natural curves in your low back and neck will keep the vertebrae in those parts from touching the floor.

3   Use your abdominal muscles to lift your pubic bone toward your chin by pulling your belly button toward your spine. Move from your sacrum first and gently flatten your low back to the floor. Proceed up your spine from there.

4   Emphasize each segment of your mid and upper back to feel the bony bumps of your vertebra press lightly into the floor—one at a time.

5   Tuck your chin to your chest and continue drawing each part of your neck back—one vertebra at a time—down.

6   Now, release the pressure and let your spine return, to its natural curve in a wave from neck to sacrum.

7   Go a bit faster and repeat for several minutes. Feel your vertebrae sequentially press and release.

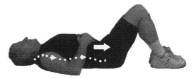 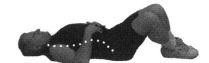 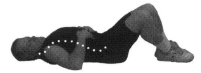

8 Add rotations or roll onto your abdomen or side to create variety. Follow whatever your body wants to do for a couple of minutes.

9 Rest and listen to the many, tiny places around your spine that are talking.

Variation #1

- ❧ Slow down your movements gradually. This will decrease your motion and momentum—and increase the use of your core muscles.

- ❧ Go as slowly as you can for five to 10 minutes.

Variation #2

- ❧ Notice how many individual vertebrae you can feel. (Remember that you have 24 plus your sacrum.)

- ❧ Try to feel a few more.

- ❧ Don't force anything in your low back or neck! If you do this undulation with the intention to feel *every* vertebra, you could hurt yourself.

As my former manager, George Evans, always told me: it's all about "Progress, not Perfection," and it's so true when it comes to the body

.

Stress Shaker

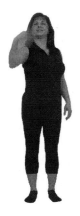 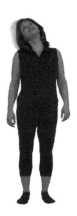 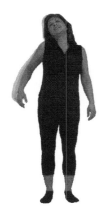

You can learn a lot about your body when you experiment with unusual movement patterns, as in this exercise. Flowing and smooth movements aren't the only beneficial ones. For some reason, I think of the comedians Steve Martin or Jerry Lewis when I do this.

1 Stand, sit, or lie down, whichever you prefer.

2 Create a twitch somewhere in your body. Maybe only a shoulder blade or buttock. Or one of your arms might take flight.

3 Rest completely.

4 Create another twitch.

5 Use all different parts of your body: arms, legs, buttocks, chest, and face. Rest momentarily after each shudder.

6 Create a twitch that includes more of your body. Use alternate combinations.

7 Flow from twitch to twitch into Free Form.

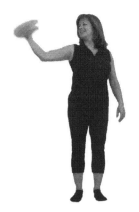 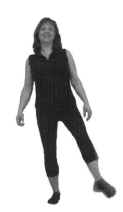 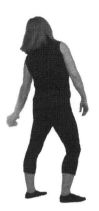

8 Feel the after-effects reverberate into every cell. Notice how much lighter and buoyant your body feels when you are rested.

Variation #1

Create a tremor by contracting and relaxing your muscles in a fast cycle.

- Once you get it started, which can take a while, keep the tremor going for 10 seconds or more.

- Try it in each arm first and then your neck and legs. This uses your deepest muscles and is a great stress reliever.

We are told to tell go of stress. But how? Send stress flying out your fingertips and surging from your skin with every twitch.

Inchworm

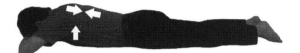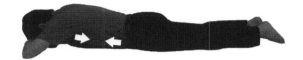

Does your back feel like one homogenous entity? Learn to manipulate the many different segments—vertebrae, ribs and individual muscles—to give yourself the dexterity of an inchworm.

1 Lie facedown on the floor with your hands under your forehead.

2 Contract your upper back muscles and drag your chest forward to create a small space between it and the floor.

3 Relax your body so that your spine is long and soft. Your torso may have inched forward along the floor ever so slightly.

4 Experiment with contracting different parts of your back. Try it in pieces and along your entire spine at once.

5 Now tighten the muscles in the front of your body to decrease the space between your pubic bone and chest. This will move your spine towards the ceiling opposite of where your muscles shorten.

6 Relax.

7 Repeat this movement, paying attention to what parts of your back move toward the ceiling. See if you can get each segment of your back to move in turn.

8 Contract your back. Relax. Contract your front. Relax. Repeat.

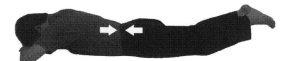 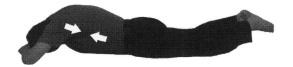

9 Use Free From to get off the ground to sitting or standing.

10 Sit and move your back and front, tiny slivers at a time. Feel your fine motor control developing.

Variation #1

❧ Inch along on your side.

Variation #2

❧ Lie on your back and imagine that you have hundred of tiny feet between you and the floor, like a millipede. Creep, using your *imaginary feet*.

As you improve your body's flexibility, you'll find it easier to go with the flow in different areas of your life.

Water Fall

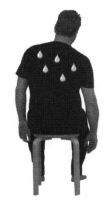 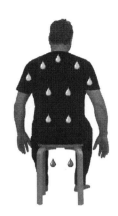 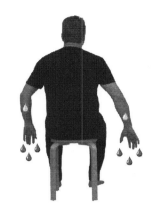

You can move as easily as water pours into a calm pool. To use less effort requires practice, but pays richly in dividends of grace and power. This exercise helped heal my neck and shoulders when a rear-end car accident left them injured and weak.

1 Sit in a chair. Let your feet and sit bones support you.

2 Slide your shoulders around and imagine a waterfall that streams over your shoulders, down your arms, and off the ends of your fingers to the floor.

3 Move as if a river ran under your skin to bathe your muscles and bones. Feel the liquid fill up your tight forearms and wrists.

4 Think of your fingers and thumbs as small water faucets. Mentally open the valves to drain the liquid from your shoulders, arms, hands, and fingers.

5 Imagine feeling water between your shoulders and neck, in that no-man's land of tension. Swish the water between your shoulder blades. Let it pour down your back, pool under your sit bones, and then spill over the seat.

6 Now feel fluid in the back of your skull. Wobble your head and let the liquid trickle down through each vertebra, to the sacrum and tailbone.

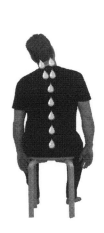 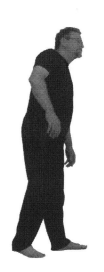 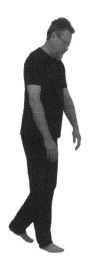

7   Enhance and expand your liquid state into a Free Form undulation for several minutes.

8   Stand or lie down. Take ownership of your fluid body.

Variation #1

ȣ Walk around and slosh like a bag full of water.

Imagine falling into soft fluffy pillows, warm water, or in love.

Undulation: Relieve Stiffness and Feel Young

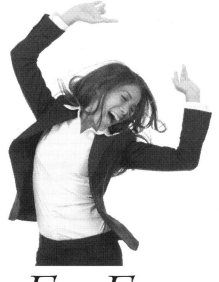

For Fun

Fun is an essential element of youthful movement. I even posit that it is central to injury-free movement. Regaining joy in movement will make everything flow more easily. I hope you are comfortable enough now with undulations to be playful, that you have enough experience with trying new movements to be able to get even more creative and adventurous with the exercises in this section.

Snake Charmer

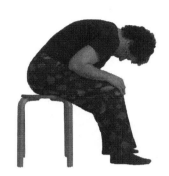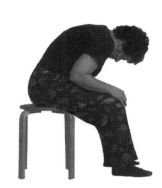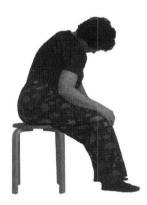

An enchanted cobra cannot resist dancing to the snake charmer's exotic notes. Mimic the beguiled and leisurely dance of the serpent with twists, turns, sways, and double-takes to improve your agility.

1   If you have Ravel's Bolero or flute music, play it.

2   Sit in a chair. Bend forward so your chest is near, or on, your thighs.

3   Arch your back; slowly raise your head and shoulders about a foot off your thighs.

4   Return to the starting position with a sideways undulation.

5   Use your hands on your thighs for support, if necessary, to give assistance to the back muscles.

6   Arch and lift, once to the right and once to the left.

7   Now rise higher and stop with your chest about two feet above your thighs. Undulate to the left and right as you wave up and down.

8   To continue, return to the start position and become the mesmerized snake uncoiling out of the basket.

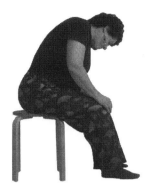 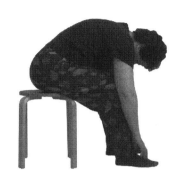 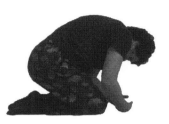

9   Stand up. Let the serpentine movements encompass your arms, legs, and entire body in a Free Form undulation.

10   Take a minute to let the flow settle into your bones.

Variation #1

Ș Kneel on a carpeted floor. Sit back on your heels or on a pillow.

Ș Fold forward so your chest is on your thighs.

Ș Undulate as above. Eventually rise up all the way so your thighs lift off the calves.

Variation #2

Ș In any position, imagine your outer skin being shed.

Ș Wriggle to be free of your skin and leave it behind.

You can accomplish more with less;
alter the old belief that all good results require hard work.

Tornado

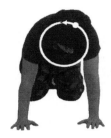 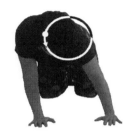 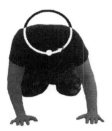

In this exercise, you'll create a funnel shape with the movement of your torso, to allow the vertebrae to twist independently. After a little practice, go ahead and work yourself into a tornado-frenzy, but please start slowly.

1 Get on your hands and knees.

2 Imagine a light shining out the crown of your head to the wall in front of you. Move your torso to draw a circle with the light.

3 Make several circles. Change directions.

4 The shape and size of the cones projected will vary, depending on the circles you draw with your chest—and how far down the spine this undulation travels.

5 Are your elbows bending as you move? Try to take the movement out of your arms; allow your ribs and shoulder blades move separately. Let your spine do the work.

6 Are your hips moving? The apex of the cone will be in your mid-back if your hips are moving directly opposite of your head. Vary the motions of your hips to make the apex travel up and down your spine.

7 To create different combinations, vary the circle direction and size and hip/neck coordination.

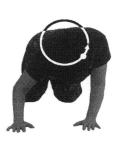 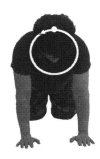 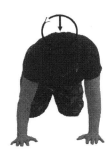

8 Transition from a Tornado into Free Form. Undulate freely for several minutes and bring your movement gently to a close.

9 Sit or lie down. Breathe, and feel your breath wave travel throughout your body.

Variation #1

- Keep your hips still as you draw circles with your head.

- This does two things. First, it requires that you use–and strengthen–your core muscles to stabilize the hips. Second, it localizes the movement to the deeper muscles around the spine.

- Change directions frequently.

Variation #2

- Start the undulation from the bottom of your spine by drawing circles with your tail.

As you try new movements, you may not feel fluid at first.
That will change with practice.

Hula Hoop

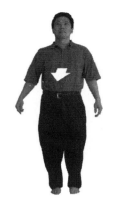 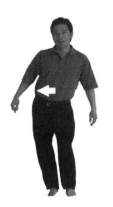 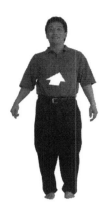

Whether or not you mastered the hula hoop as a child, your spine will benefit if you pretend to swing one around your middle in a constant and balanced motion. Extend the circular motion down to your hips and your love life will thank you as well.

1   Stand comfortably.

2   Trace a figurative circle around your middle, at the level of your belly button, to get a tactile sense of where a hula hoop would rest.

3   Keep your feet in place and move your belly around in this order: forward, right, back, left, and forward again.

4   Smooth out the corners and make circles, five clockwise and five counter-clockwise.

5   Make your chest the epicenter of the motion. Repeat five times each direction.

6   Now draw circles with your hips, five times each direction.

7   Widen your stance and turn your circles into a dance. Dance Free Form for several minutes.

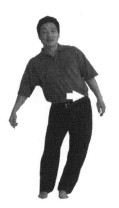 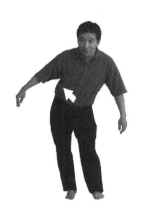 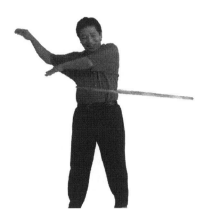

8 Rest for a minute. See if you can maintain the lively energy in your middle, but remain calm in your limbs and focused in your head.

Variation #1

∿ In order, circle your chest, belly button, and hips—one circle with each moving up and down your body.

Variation #2

∿ Get a real hula hoop. Concentrate on the forward and back motions, and it's actually easier to keep the hula hooping.

Make it fun.

Partners

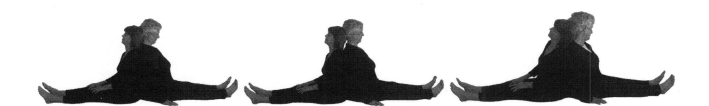

Here's an opportunity to share and deepen your undulation experience. By now, you've probably aroused the curiosity of others in your life, with all the wiggling and giggling, and the resulting grace. Enlist one of them to help—and benefit from the fluidity of motion.

1 Sit back to back, on the floor or straddling a bench. Get comfortable.

2 Notice each other's backs for a moment—where you touch, the spaces between, the curves, and the movement of breath.

3 Ask your partner to follow your lead through slow sways, twists, turns, and waves. Try to maintain consistent contact.

4 Be sensitive and undulate within your partner's abilities for a couple of minutes.

5 Now ask your partner to lead. Assure her that nothing has to be choreographed or similar to how you led the movement.

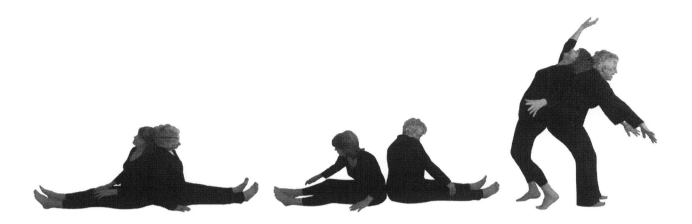

6 Break away from each other and undulate separately. Let your bodies be free.

7 Rest for a minute with your back to a wall.

Variation #1

❧ Stand back to back and take turns leading the undulations. Do your best to stay in contact.

Look to nature for inspiration: fields of grain,
sprouting seeds, rippling creeks, stalking tigers.

Appendix 1: Exercises Alphabetically

Appendix 2: Exercises by Category

Bibliography

Anderson, Bob. *Stretching*. Bolinas, CA: Shelter Publications, 2000.

Barral, Jean-Pierre, Mercier, Pierre. *Visceral Manipulation*. Seattle, WA: Eastland Press, 1988.

Butler, Sharon J. *Conquering Carpal Tunnel Syndrome*. Oakland, CA: New Harbinger Publications, 1996.

Calais-Germain, Blandine. *Anatomy of Movement*. Seattle, Washington: Eastland Press, 1993.

Centers for Disease Control, National Center for Health Statistics, "The National Nursing Home Survey" 1999 Summary.

Chikly, M.D., D.O. (hon.), Bruno. *Theory and Practice of Lymph Drainage Therapy* 2nd Edition. Scottsdale, AZ: I.H.H. Publishing, 2004.

Conrad, Emilie and Valarie Hunt. *Life on Land: The Story of Continuum and the World Renowned Self-Discovery and Movement Method*. Berkeley, CA: North Atlantic Books, 2007.

Ellis, William, Polynesian Researches, 1859, New Zealand Texts Collection

Farhi, Donna. *Yoga Mind Body & Spirit*. New York, NY: Henry Holt and Company, 2000.

Foster, Mary Ann. *Somatic Patterning*. Longmont, CO: EMS Press, 2004.

Franklin, Eric. *Dynamic Alignment Through Imagery*. Champaign, IL: Human Kinetics, 1996.

Gray's Anatomy, 38th Edition. London, England: Churchill Livingstone, 1995, reprint 1999.

Hackney, Peggy. *Making Connections Total Body Integration Through Bartenieff Fundamentals*. New York, NY: Routledge, 2002.

Heller, Joseph and William A.Henkin. *Bodywise*. Berkeley, CA: North Atlantic Books, 2004.

Hellerwork Client Handbook. Mt. Shasta, CA: Hellerwork International, 2005.

Herzog, Walter and Benno M. Nigg (editors). *Biomechanics of the Muscolo-Skeletal Sytem*, Second Edition. West Sussex, England: John Wiley & Son, Ltd., 1999, reprint 2005.

Kendall, P.T., F.A.P.T.A., Florence Peterson, et al. *Muscles Testing and Function*. Baltimore, MD: Williams & Wilkins, 1993.

Kraftsow, Gary. *Yoga for Wellness*. New York, NY: Penguin Putnam, 1999.

Myers, Thomas W. *Anatomy Trains*. Edinburgh, England: Churchill Livingston, 2001.

Netter, MD, Frank H. *Atlas of Human Anatomy*. East Hanover, NJ: Novartis1989, second edition 1997.

Rolf, Ph.D., Ida P., *Rolfing®: Reestablishing the Natural Alignment and Structural Integration of the Human Body for Vitality and Well-*

Being. Rochester, VT: Healing Arts Press, 1989.

Sahrmann, Ph.D., PT, FATA, Shirley. *Diagnosis and Treatment of Movement Impairment Syndromes.* St. Louis, MI: Mosby, 2002.

Schultz, Ph. D. R. Louis and Rosemary Feitis, D.O. *The Endless Web.* Berkeley, CA: North Atlantic Books, 1996.

Simon, M.D., Harvey B. *The No Sweat Exercise Plan.* New York, NY: McGraw Hill, 2006.

Theodosakis, M.D., M.S., M.P.H, Jason, et al. *Maximizing the Arthritis Cure.* New York, NY: St. Martin's Press, 1998.

Travell, M.D., Janet G. and David G. Simmons, M.D. *Myofascial Pain and Dysfunction: The Trigger Point Manual Volume I.* Baltimore, MD: Williams & Wilkins, 1983.

Upledger DO FAAO, John E. and Jon D. Vredevoogd, MFA. *Craniosacral Therapy.* Seattle, WA: Eastland Press, 1983.

Exercises

You will find undulation exercises from many sources, therefore some of the exercises may be similar to those you and I have tried in yoga or other modalities. Most of the exercises in this book, as they are written, were developed by me as I undulated in my home. However, a few are adaptations of specific exercises I have found elsewhere. They are:

- ∞ Snake Arms, variation #2 is adapted from *Conquering Carpal Tunnel Syndrome* by Sharon Butler.

- ∞ Breathing, is similar to a combination of exercises found in *Yoga Mind Body & Spirit* by Donna Farhi.

- ∞ Train Cars, is an adaptation of Yield & Push Pattern from Head and Tail from *Making Connections by Peggy Hackney.*

- ∞ Eric Franklin's *Dynamic Alignment Through Imagery* includes many sensory-rich exercises including a Pelvic Geyser and Foot Dome with waterspout which inspired *Fountain.*

About the Author

Anita Boser

Anita did not invent undulation, but she created a way to make this fundamental movement pattern accessible to people who don't move well. As a Certified Hellerwork Practitioner and Board Certified Structural Integrator℠, she helps her clients regain their fluidity, alignment, and vitality with a combination of bodywork, awareness dialogue, and movement education. Her specialty is teaching people how to use small movements to melt stuck places in their bodies, especially in the back.

In addition to her profession and daily undulation, she is experienced in belly dancing, yoga, and karate, all of which have helped her develop a variety of exercises that transform bodies from stiff and uncomfortable to graceful and at ease.

Anita believes that having fun is essential to enjoying life, a lesson she learned from her husband, Michael, and twin sons, Jeff and Ryan, who keep her laughing on a regular basis.